How To Cope With Asthma And Hay Fever

A Complete Guide

by
Graham Jones

IMPERIA BOOKS LIMITED

First published 1994
by Imperia Books Ltd.
© 1994 Graham Jones

British Library Cataloguing
in Publication Data.
A catalogue record for this book
is available from the British Library.

IBSN 1 897656 06 8

Cover by Sarah Davies
Typeset by Carter Wordsmiths, London

Published by
IMPERIA BOOKS LIMITED
Canada House, Blackburn Road, London NW6 1RZ

Printed in Great Britain by Black Bear Press Ltd., Cambridge

Foreword

by Dr Dan Williams MB BCh,
partner in a busy London group practice
which runs an Asthma Clinic as part of its services.

This clear and well informed book will be welcomed by the growing population of asthma and hay fever sufferers. It will also appeal to a wider audience and help to reassure those people who think that they may be suffering from these conditions but have not yet sought medical help.

It presents important information on the scientific basis for asthma and allergic conditions and their treatment, as well as exploring alternative approaches.

In today's general practice setting, the average consultation is often too short to give patients with asthma or hay fever the time they really need to understand their condition. Too often, they are frightened by the diagnosis and leave the surgery filled with anxiety and unanswered questions. Community-based asthma clinics go a long way towards addressing this problem.

This readable and reader-friendly book will provide a welcome source of reference for millions of sufferers. It can be recommended with confidence by the professionals who look after them.

Dan Williams

Contents

Introduction

Asthma and hay fever are frighteningly common. Together they affect nine million people in the UK alone – that's one person in every six! Asthma is particularly common in children, affecting 15% of all youngsters. In the average school class, for instance, there will be four or five children who suffer from this potentially fatal condition. Meanwhile, hay fever afflicts one person in every nine.

If you work in an average business with around 50 employees, you would be working alongside six hay fever sufferers and three people with asthma. Large high street banks, for instance, employ around 100,000 people. That means that there are probably around 5,000 people with asthma working for any one of them; and a further 11,000 of its staff suffer from hay fever.

Added to that, £1m is spent every day in the UK on asthma drugs; and in a city like Birmingham, 150 people a week are admitted to hospital with an asthma attack.

Six people die from asthma every day – a figure that hasn't changed since records began, in spite of improved treatment. Worryingly, there is also evidence that the recorded figure of 2,000 asthma deaths a year may be rising.

As if all these statistics were not bad enough, researchers believe that the actual figures may be worse. They think that as many as 50% of children with asthma are not diagnosed as having the condition.

Clearly, hay fever and asthma are major health problems. There is no doubt that you will know at least someone who suffers from one of them; and the chances of you not knowing anyone with either condition are slim in the extreme.

This book is aimed at every one of the nine million people with asthma or hay fever. But because there are millions of children who have asthma or hay fever, this book is also particularly suitable for their parents. Whether you are a parent or a sufferer yourself, this book will give you a complete guide to coping with either of these conditions and will help you or your child live as near normal a life as possible.

The following pages contain numerous practical hints and tips on coping with asthma or hay fever. They will be particularly useful if you are one of the three quarters of a million people who unfortunately suffer from both these complaints.

The book is arranged in short sections, allowing you to dip in and out of topics as you want. You do not have to read it from cover to cover, though you will obviously gain much more if you do so. If you don't want to read the entire book straight away, Chapter 12 provides a complete plan for looking after yourself if you are a sufferer, as well as a practical guide for parents of children with asthma or hay fever.

But however you approach these conditions, you will find that the seriousness of these common health problems is emphasised throughout the book. You should always seek medical advice which takes your own individual circumstances into account. This book can help – but it should not be taken as the complete answer for every case. It is intended to be supplementary to the medical advice you receive; but even so, you should find it very useful.

Chapter 1
About Asthma

An asthma attack is one of the most frightening experiences any of us can suffer. It is also a most traumatic happening to watch. You feel helpless. The victim is clearly suffering badly and yet there is little you can do to help. An asthma attack is a living nightmare for everyone involved.

Sally's story

Sally, aged 19 and a student of foreign languages, was diagnosed as suffering from asthma when she was six years old. She has had many attacks over the years but, with the help of her doctor, has managed to keep her asthma in check – though she knows it will never go away.

Last March she was walking the mile and a half from her bed-sit to the university on a cold and muggy day. It was 8.45 am, the middle of the morning rush of cars taking kids to school and people to work.

Sally noticed that her chest felt a little tighter than normal. After about a mile, she was forced to stop, take a rest and use her inhaler to top-up her medication. Sally waited for a while and then went on to the first lecture of the day which she didn't want to miss. It was important as her exams were due at the end of the term, just before Easter.

Sally needed some more medication during the lectures as her chest still felt tight. She started to worry that she was going to have an attack; and her chest began to tighten even more. She went outside during the morning break, but the cold morning air took her breath away and she needed more medication to keep her going. By lunch time, Sally had been admitted to hospital.

In her own words:

It all happened so suddenly. It was just like being a small child again. I thought I had got over these bad attacks; but the cold air, the walk through the traffic and the stress of coming up to exams all took their toll I'm afraid – and, whoosh, there I was kneeling on the ground outside the lecture theatre, gasping for air.

She added:

Having an asthma attack is hard to describe. It's like no other experience.
To me, it feels as though there is someone inside my chest squeezing my lungs and stopping me from breathing. You try as hard as you can to get air into your lungs – but they just won't take it. No matter how hard you try to breathe in, nothing seems to happen. You gasp for air, desperate to get some oxygen into your lungs, and still it won't get in. It's like trying to take deep breaths through a straw.

Sally's friend Angela, the girl who called the ambulance and got her to hospital, was terrified by the incident.

I have never seen anything like it. It was really very distressing.
Sally was literally clawing the air around her, trying to get air towards her. She looked a sort of grey colour and you could see the sheer panic in her eyes. I thought at one point she was going to die.
And I felt so stupid – I just didn't know what to do to help her. She couldn't breathe properly and there was nothing I could do, except to stroke her hair away from her face and say the ambulance was on its way. How stupid that seems now.

Sally's attack led to three days in hospital, some injections of a powerful drug and the realisation that she will never be safe from attack.

For Angela, the incident showed her the seriousness of asthma. Before then, she had thought that sufferers relied on their inhalers almost as a psychological prop. Now she knows better.

Asthma people

People like Sally and Angela are not rare. Asthma attacks are serious, frightening and worrying events. Those who witness them feel helpless and stupid. Those who suffer them feel a state of panic and wonder if they will survive.

A few years ago, an educational initiative, Action Asthma, carried out an important survey of asthma in the UK. Following that survey, the organisation revealed some of the thoughts of asthma patients.

• One 45 year old woman with a 30 year history of asthma said:

To have asthma means that you have to struggle for every breath you take. It feels as if someone is holding your head under water and you are going to drown.

My life has been spent in and out of hospitals and in bed at home for long periods on massive doses of steroids. I have been unable to work now for 12 years.

- A 52 year old man said:

I have had asthma since I was two years old. It has affected me for almost all my life. All decisions have to be taken with asthma in mind.

- A 65 year old woman, who had only recently been diagnosed as having asthma, said:

It is very easy for someone with asthma to be written off as not much fun. But all the sufferer is quietly trying to do at the party or the dance is to breathe.

But other kinds of people also have asthma.

- Adrian Moorhouse, the Olympic swimmer, for instance, has suffered from asthma since he was seven years old. Yet by the age of 14 he was competing nationally. He later represented Britain in the Los Angeles Olympics in 1984 and in the Seoul games in 1988, where he won a Gold medal for the 100m breaststroke.

- Alan Pascoe, who suffered from asthma, competed in the 1972 Munich Olympics where he won a silver medal in the 4x400m relay race. He also competed in the Montreal Olympics in 1976. Alan Pascoe holds a number of gold medals for hurdling in world games and championships.

Clearly, asthma is not a hindrance for some people. It is faced as a serious condition – but handled properly to make exemplary physical performance possible. For other people, as the Action Asthma survey showed, asthma is a real problem which makes life difficult to cope with.

But what people like the old lady at the dance, struggling for breath, and someone like Adrian Moorhouse have in common is the fact that asthma symptoms need to be dealt with. Although many sportsmen and sports-women have asthma, their condition doesn't go away because they are fit athletes. They still have to cope with their symptoms and with possible attacks.

3

Asthma symptoms

People often do not notice asthma symptoms at the early stages of the disease, before their first attack takes them to their doctor. Since a considerable number of first attacks are experienced in children, their onset can be really worrying for parents. However, there are usually some signs of asthma being present, well before an attack happens.

Wheezing is usually the first sign. The breathing pattern becomes noisier than usual and you can hear air vibrating in the lungs. With asthma, the noise is most often worst when the victim is attempting to breathe out. Another common sign of asthma is a persistent cough. This usually becomes worse with exercise and is often particularly troublesome at night. The cough is usually mild and sometimes disappears altogether in the afternoons.

These are not the only symptoms of asthma. The wheezing may become so troublesome that the sufferer gets worried. That can lead to symptoms of anxiety – such as sweating, a rapid heart rate and, curiously enough, an attempt to breathe even faster. Thus a vicious circle begins. But whatever else happens, patients with asthma invariably describe tightness around the chest – as though a belt is being tightened around the rib cage, restricting the lungs.

The lungs

The first thing that happens in asthma is the inflammation of the airways leading through the lungs. These airways are responsible for delivering the air we breathe into direct contact with our bloodstream – so that life-giving oxygen can be transferred into the blood and poisonous gases, like carbon dioxide, can be removed from the blood and breathed out.

The airways are a complex series of tubes and pipes that go from very large to microscopically small. The windpipe is the largest tube in the airways – about an inch in diameter and five inches long. This divides into two smaller tubes just above the heart, one for each lung. These then divide down again into smaller tubes; and the smaller tubes divide again and again into ever smaller ones. The tiniest tubes in the system are less than a millimetre wide.

In asthma, all the tubes of the airways can become inflamed and filled with phlegm – which restricts the passage of air through them. The result

4

is seen in increasingly futile attempts to take deep breaths – ineffective because the tubes are so inflamed that little air can get through.

The process of asthma

A number of other biological reactions begin once the lungs have become inflamed.

The muscles in the walls of the airway tubes start to contract and reduce the size of the tubes. In combination with the inflammation and the release of phlegm, that makes the condition worse and diminishes the amount of air an asthma sufferer can breathe in and out.

If you have asthma, or if your child suffers from it, you will soon get used to doctors talking about the measurement of the amount of air that goes in and out of the lungs.

The air that goes in and out at each breath is known as the tidal volume. This amounts to about half a litre of air in healthy individuals; but is only a tiny proportion of the five or six litres of air that the lungs of a normal adult male can hold.

When breathing out, a normal adult male can usually exhale about three and a half litres of air in the first second – that is at a rate of about 600 litres per minute.

All these measurements are very much reduced for people with asthma. The amount of air breathed out in a second, known as the Forced Expiratory Volume (FEV), is often very low. The rate at which the air flows, the Peak Expiratory Flow (PEF), is also reduced and may be as low as 200 litres per minute – only a third as effective as in a normal individual.

Both these measurements are used a great deal in the diagnosis and management of people with asthma; and many sufferers take their own PEF measurements regularly with a device provided by their doctor on prescription.

What these measurements demonstrate is that people with asthma have lungs which are relatively inefficient in moving air in and out again. That's due entirely to the narrowing of the airways.

Suppose you are due to water the garden with a hose pipe attached to the kitchen tap. Like other hose pipes it's about an inch in diameter and you are able to water the garden fairly well with it in just a few minutes. Now imagine that the pipe attached to your tap has been flattened by someone placing heavy objects along its length. The water can still get through, but only just. How long will it now take to water your garden with the flow reduced to a trickle? You can still do the job but it will take a lot longer.

That's what happens in asthma; the airways have been narrowed by inflammation, muscular contraction and the production of phlegm. The lungs can still be used for breathing – but it's far more difficult than if the tubes were wide open.

Diagnosing asthma

A check-up with your GP is necessary if you suspect asthma in yourself or in your child.

You may have had symptoms of wheezing or a persistent cough. You might also have woken in the night to find it hard to breathe. Anything to do with your breathing must be reported to give the doctor a full picture of what is happening.

Also, tell your doctor if the symptoms occur at particular times of day, in specific places or after certain meals.

The doctor will need to examine you. This will first involve listening to your lungs through a stethoscope, which amplifies the noises in your chest and allows the doctor to hear what is going on inside the lungs. The stethoscope will be used on your front and on your back. The doctor will spend some time listening to your lungs. You will be asked to breathe normally, take in deep breaths, breathe out deeply, breathe slowly as well as cough. You might even be asked to speak, particularly to say "ninety nine". That sounds daft, but the words "ninety nine" are particularly useful in making your lungs vibrate.

Having listened to your lungs through a stethoscope, the doctor will then want to tap your chest. This is done using a technique known as percussion. The doctor places two fingers against your chest and then taps them with two fingers of the other hand. The lungs are healthy if a hollow sound is produced; but a dull noise indicates that the lungs have fluid in them – usually due to some kind of inflammation.

Usually, these tests and your description of the symptoms will be enough for a doctor to diagnose asthma. In fact, many cases can be identified simply from the description of the patient's symptoms. However, sometimes the doctor may not be quite sure, or may want to eliminate other causes of the symptoms, before confirming asthma as the diagnosis. You may also be referred to the local chest clinic for further examination and tests.

A blood test may be taken and a chest X-ray. For most asthma sufferers, their chest X-rays look perfectly normal and doctors only order them to eliminate other potential causes of the symptoms – such as infections or, in young children, cystic fibrosis.

You will most likely be asked to undergo a number of lung function tests – the Forced Expiratory Volume (FEV) test and the Peak Expiratory Flow (PEF) test (see page 5). Every GP nowadays has a small hand-held machine that is highly effective in determining the efficiency of your lungs. The machinery needed for testing FEV is more complex and is usually only available in hospitals.

The other tests your doctor may suggest are those to identify the particular things that trigger attacks. If symptoms only seem to come on at work and you are an assistant at a local cattery, this might make the doctor suspect that you are allergic to animal fur. An allergy test would help confirm this.

Allergy tests are straightforward. A drop of liquid containing the suspected problem substance is placed on your arm. Then a small pinprick is made through the liquid into the skin. If you are allergic to the substance, the area around the pinprick becomes inflamed and itchy.

Food allergies

Particular foods can affect people with asthma.

It is often difficult to detect the culprit in a range of possible foods, as it may well be that someone has an allergy to a specific component in food or to one particular food additive. It may not be so simple as finding that shellfish, for instance, cause the problem.

Testing for food allergy

An allergic reaction to food is rarely immediate and often comes on some hours after eating. Food stays in the digestive system for two to three days – so you may suffer symptoms quite a while after eating the problem substance.

It's a good idea to consider the possibility of a food allergy if you cannot find what in particular triggers attacks of symptoms. Indeed, many people with asthma discover that particular foods make them far more susceptible to whatever it is that triggers their attacks.

The first thing to do is to keep a diary. Note down the contents of each meal; and also keep a record of episodes of wheeziness and asthma attacks. You'll need to keep this up for about a month or so to get a true record of your eating patterns and symptoms.

By looking back over it, you may then be able to spot a common pattern. For instance, you may find that you developed symptoms each day after eating sausages. But only by keeping a written record of your meals and your symptoms will the link become obvious.

Another thing to do is to keep a record of your pulse rate. This is best felt in the wrist; use the first two fingers of your other hand to check it. Never use your thumb as this also has a pulse in it and you will get a wrong result. Count the number of beats in a minute.

Sit down and relax for a few minutes before every meal: then take your pulse and make a note of it. Ensure that you don't do any vigorous exercise for about 15 to 30 minutes after the meal; and then take your pulse again – but only after you have been sitting down relaxed for a couple of minutes. If the pulse rate has increased by more than about ten beats per minute, you are probably allergic to something you have eaten.

A further way of testing for food allergies is to adapt your diet. Let someone else prepare a meal for you so that you don't know what is in it – foods thought to be allergic should be disguised in some way so that you do not develop symptoms as a result of a psychological reaction. If you do develop symptoms, without knowing that you have eaten an offending food, this will confirm that you are indeed allergic to it.

However, many people do not find it easy to discover which food is responsible. Their diary does not point to any particular culprits and symptoms occur after eating a wide range of foods. For them, a special programme of eating, known as an exclusion diet, is the best way forward.

Exclusion diets

These work by cutting out all foods to which you think you might be allergic and then gradually introducing possible culprits, one by one.

Ideally, you shouldn't eat a thing for about five days – but that's rarely practicable. So eat a very narrow range of foods that you are pretty sure do not seem to cause any trouble. Exclude all dairy products completely – no milk, butter, cheese, etc.

Eat your narrow diet for about ten days and then add in the possible problem foods, one at a time. Keep a record of what you eat and your symptoms. You will be able to identify the problem foods as symptoms will develop quite soon after you have eaten them.

An exclusion diet is a tedious and time consuming process; but it is often the only way to find out which specific food is causing the problem.

What the diagnosis will mean

The results of medical tests and exclusion diets, combined with the information you give your doctor, will lead to the eventual diagnosis.

If it is asthma, and the specific cause has been identified by the tests, the doctor will then discuss the various treatment options with you. Even if the specific cause hasn't yet been identified, the doctor will still want to treat your symptoms; but may also suggest further tests to find out exactly what causes the problem in your case.

But don't worry if it is asthma. Being labelled as asthmatic may sound like a stigma; but having asthma doesn't mean your life will be ruined. True, life with asthma will not be easy; but neither should living a normal life be impossible – providing you treat the condition seriously. Always remember that asthma is potentially life threatening.

Other allergies

People with asthma may be allergic to things other than food.

One of the most common is animal fur. It is hardly worthwhile testing for allergy to animal fur if attacks always follow contact with a pet. Attacks can follow stroking a cat, for instance. If this does occur, it is usually a sign that the allergy is to animal fur; and you will experience a dramatic improvement in your condition if you keep well out of the way of animals. For parents of youngsters with asthma this often means getting rid of the dog or the cat.

Chronic asthma

In some cases the diagnosis may be chronic asthma. This serious and highly troubling type of asthma affects about one in every hundred people with asthma.

They are breathless for much of the time; and even small amounts of exertion can bring on bad episodes of wheeziness. It is particularly common in middle aged people and the elderly, but can also occur in children. Chronic asthma can be very worrying because of the periods of breathlessness which accompany the wheezing.

Doctors treat chronic asthma very seriously and prescribe the strongest treatments possible to control the symptoms. Even so, many people with chronic asthma do find their lifestyles severely restricted because of breathlessness.

The problem of asthma

Asthma is a serious condition. Though its diagnosis is relatively straightforward, doctors are often cautious about confirming it until they have done a battery of tests. The reason is that labelling someone as asthmatic will have an impact on the rest of his or her life. Doctors are therefore reluctant to say you have asthma until they are absolutely sure.

This is a two-sided problem. It means that some people with mild asthma probably go untreated for a while because of the fear of labelling them asthmatic. It also means that in many cases, true asthma sufferers are forced to wait for effective treatment while all the test results are being awaited.

Your doctor may be cautious about making a diagnosis of asthma when you first pop along to the surgery. The answer is to be persistent and to ensure that he or she knows absolutely everything about your symptoms. Don't leave anything out, no matter how trivial you may think it is. A diagnosis is much more easily made if your doctor is well informed.

A difficulty with some asthma sufferers is that they often don't tell the doctor enough in the first instance. They then risk the chance of going without proper treatment for a while – and that cannot be good for them.

Chapter 2
About Hay Fever

Hay fever is always caused by a particular agent that triggers the body's defence mechanisms into action. At first sight this looks easy to counter. If all you have to do is to work out which particular substance is responsible for your symptoms, preventing hay fever would be simple.

Sadly, this is not the picture that most people with hay fever will understand. Apart from the fact that there are many different things that can cause attacks of symptoms, there is another problem. People with hay fever can respond to one cause one year, and to a different one the following year. Hay fever isn't static. For example, a particular pollen may be plentiful one year and rare the next because the trees that brought the pollens in the first year have been chopped down. So the things that trigger an attack of symptoms of hay fever can vary considerably.

For this reason, people with hay fever often give up trying to find the actual cause of their symptoms. Instead, they try to deal with the symptoms themselves and only worry about the cause if it results in a really drastic problem.

Even so, life is not that easy. Dealing with the symptoms can be a significant battle in itself; for hay fever is often much more than just a runny nose. Indeed, almost one million working days are lost in the UK each year as a result of hay fever.

Doreen's story

Doreen is 64 and lives with her husband in a cottage in the West Country. She has lived in the area all her life and, although she has now retired, used to work in the village shop.

Six years ago, she was on her way to work on a fine early morning in May. The sun was shining. It was warm and she was really enjoying the walk down the street towards the shop. She remembers waving to one of the local farm workers passing by. Other than that, it appeared to be an uneventful stroll to the shop.

Later that morning though, Doreen began to feel strange. She developed a mild headache and felt as if she was going to get a cold. She remembers sneezing a few times and developing a runny nose. At first, she thought it was just an annoying summer cold. Later that afternoon, her eyes began to itch and her throat felt raw. She thought it was going to be a very nasty cold. Within two days, her stroll to work had become a terrible experience. In her own words:

I just didn't know what was happening. The ten minute stroll down through the village was the start of something quite awful. My eyes were streaming and itching dreadfully. My throat felt dry and I developed a nasty, wheezy cough. I also had a nose that seemed to pour. I really thought I was becoming seriously ill.

Within a week, Doreen had given up her job. She found that the symptoms were less severe if she remained indoors at home just outside the village. She still got attacks of the symptoms once or twice a day – but nothing like as badly as on the walk to work in the mornings. One day, for instance, she thought she was really very ill because her eyes started to puff up and she looked like she'd been three rounds with Frank Bruno!

Her doctor quickly diagnosed hay fever. Doreen thought it was more serious as she had never suffered before from this condition. Her doctor explained that anyone can get hay fever at any time of life.

Later she discovered that she was allergic to hawthorn which releases its pollen during the spring and early summer. She realised for the first time just how many hawthorn bushes there are in the village hedgerows.

Hay fever people

Doreen's story is not untypical. People are forced to give up careers, find new jobs or even move house because of hay fever.

Take the example of Alan who is 34 years old and lives on the edge of a small town in Hampshire. He works from home as a computer consultant and spends part of his time there and the other part visiting clients.

Behind his house is a field which was formerly used for wheat production. Because of a government scheme to ensure that farmers do not overproduce, the field has now been set-aside and is no longer used to grow crops. Instead, grasses and plants grow wild there.

Alan noticed that something was different during the first summer after the set-aside came into operation. He explained:

I noticed that when I was at home during the summer my skin became very itchy and my nose started to run. At first, I thought I was coming down with some dreadful disease. However, the symptoms quickly disappeared when I was away from the house with a client. I began to think there was something wrong with my house.

Alan saw his doctor and was told that the symptoms were like those of hay fever. He was given some treatment and told not to worry. Alan decided not to take the treatment – he dislikes medicines and only takes tablets when he is really ill.

However, soon he realised he no longer needed the treatment, for his itching had subsided and his nose was back to normal. That coincided with the field returning to a blanket of green; and Alan concluded that his symptoms only occurred when there were weeds with white heads in the field. The pollen released by those weeds had triggered his symptoms.

But Alan's work had been badly affected by his experience. He said:

When I was at home, I just couldn't concentrate. The itching and the runny nose meant that I was stopping work every five minutes. It took me four times as long as it should have done to achieve things.

I discovered that living on the edge of the countryside was great for the view, but no good for helping to pay the mortgage.

Alan's house is now up for sale; and he is hoping to move away from fields with pollinating weeds. Only in that way can he carry on working uninterrupted and keep his clients happy.

The point of Alan's story is that, like Doreen, hay fever caused a change in his life. He needed to move house; and Doreen had to give up her job. Hay fever is not just a sniffle and a sneeze. It alters the lives of many sufferers. Indeed for some, hay fever symptoms are so bad during the summer that they are trapped in their homes, with windows and doors firmly shut to keep as much pollen out as possible – prisoners of hay fever.

Hay fever seasons

There are three principal times of the year when hay fever occurs – spring, early summer and late summer. Each time brings different pollens. The spring is when most trees pollinate, so trouble then is often due to trees. The early summer brings grass pollens and there are over 10,000 of them to cope with. The late summer brings hay fever induced by flower and weed pollens. These are the broad categories. You can be affected by different pollens at any time of the year; but the three main seasons are when the most likely pollens to affect sufferers are released.

You cannot put a definite time on pollens. Trees do not know that it's April 15th – and therefore it's pollen release day! Pollination varies due to factors including the weather, pollution, the amount of sunshine, the dryness or wetness of the year and a myriad of other reasons. This means that trees may start pollinating in March one year and in February or even May the following year. You can't be sure. What you can be sure of is that the amount of pollen in the air is going to be high on a humid summer morning.

Pollen counts

Symptoms are at their worst when the pollen count is high. The pollen count is a measure of the number of pollen particles in the air you breathe. The more pollen in the air, the more likely you are to have symptoms. As the pollen count rises, symptoms will worsen. In the UK pollen counts are mostly measured in June and July, the worst months for hay fever sufferers.

To measure the pollen count – which is the number of pollen particles in a cubic metre of air – the Meteorological Office uses special devices that encourage pollen particles to stick to sheets of glass coated with a sticky material. The glass is then examined under a microscope and the amount of pollen calculated.

The pollen count is graded into three levels. A low pollen count is when there are fewer than 4,000 particles of pollen in each cubic metre of air. If the number is between 4,000 and 5,000, the pollen count is described as moderate. It is a high pollen count when the number exceeds 5,000; and you can be sure that symptoms will be at their worst.

Hay fever symptoms

The symptoms of hay fever vary. For some people it is simply a runny nose; for others it is more like an attack of flu. The symptoms also vary for each individual sufferer from time to time. The nose may be affected at one season and the eyes at another.

Hay fever affects the upper respiratory tract. This is the part of the breathing apparatus that comes before the windpipe – the nose, the pharynx (the system behind the nose) and the throat.

Pollen is very quickly absorbed when breathed in – for the nose, pharynx and throat all have a very rich blood supply, close to the surface. Pollens therefore have an easy route into the blood, where they cause an almost instantaneous reaction – inflammation and the release of fluids. Because the reaction is quick and localised, the results are also local with the inflammation and the fluid release all occurring in the nose, the pharynx and the throat.

Inflammation and fluid release in the nose leads to the usual symptoms of many hay fever sufferers – a runny nose accompanied by sneezing. If the pollen gets further back into the throat, there can be coughing and wheezing, almost like asthma symptoms. The throat becomes sore and headaches can occur.

Pollen affects the eyes of some sufferers. This is because the soft tissues around the eyes also have a rich blood supply, very close to the surface, which quickly absorbs pollen blown onto the eyelids by the wind. That leads to eye inflammation – redness, swelling and watering. People with hay fever often have streaming eyes.

Diagnosing hay fever

The diagnosis of hay fever is not difficult. Someone walking into the doctor's surgery with red eyes, sneezing, and with hanky in hand, is almost certain to have hay fever – if it is spring or summer. Flu and colds are more usually winter conditions.

When asked to describe your symptoms, you should give the doctor as full a description as possible, saying when symptoms are at their worst. You'll probably find they are at their most awful in the afternoons. Make sure you talk about every symptom, no matter how trivial. There are a few conditions that can mimic hay fever and your doctor will want to exclude these. Most importantly your doctor will want to exclude a condition known as drug-induced rhinitis, which leads to symptoms of hay fever in patients taking particular medicines.

All sorts of drugs can also cause hay fever symptoms, including those that treat blood pressure, antibiotics, sleeping pills, tranquillisers and even aspirin.

Also, hay fever symptoms can be brought on by contact with some industrial chemicals; and so your GP will need to know details of your occupation if you work in any kind of business where chemicals are used. They, and not pollen, may be responsible for the symptoms.

If your doctor does suspect hay fever, you might be asked to undergo some tests. The usual test is one to determine which pollen is causing the difficulty. A series of drops of liquid are placed on your forearm, each containing different pollen allergens. Then small pinpricks are made into the skin through the liquid, allowing it to come into contact with your blood. The area becomes red and inflamed if you are susceptible to one of the allergens.

Unfortunately, this kind of testing can be a bit hit and miss for there are thousands of different pollens; and to be tested for allergy against all of them would take many months. You may sometimes continue to get symptoms even though the specific pollen hasn't been identified in a whole batch of tests. Doctors usually then give up the tests because it's better to get rid of your symptoms than to go on trying to find the specific culprit causing the problem. So, testing is often not carried out at all on most patients and is reserved for people with the severest symptoms.

Newer diagnostic techniques are now being introduced for those with really disabling symptoms. These include special fibre-optic tubes that can be inserted into the nasal passages to give the specialist a clear view of what is happening inside them. Special X-ray style imaging techniques are also becoming available to identify exactly what is going on. However, such techniques are rarely used for ordinary patients.

The problem with hay fever

Most people can easily identify the symptoms of hay fever. Indeed many obtain remedies directly from their local chemist and do not even trouble their doctor.

A major problem with hay fever is the time of year at which it first occurs. Most symptoms begin in spring and early summer – and that's just when schools and colleges hold examinations. It's also when people try to relax and take a summer holiday. You simply cannot perform well in exams if you are sneezing, have itchy eyes and a sore throat. Equally you can hardly enjoy a summer break if you are forever blowing your nose, wheezing and having to avoid being in the open air.

Unlike asthma, where the condition is expected to affect sufferers more seriously, hay fever is often regarded as trivial. Teachers, bosses and colleagues will expect you to soldier on, even though you feel like curling up in bed and taking something to put you to sleep for a day or two. Unfortunately, that is seldom possible and you just have to cope as best you can. With hay fever it is often difficult to get people to accept that you are unwell.

Happily, there is a way out; and that is to be up front about your condition. Tell people you suffer from hay fever and describe how you feel – particularly to bosses and schoolteachers. Attempting to hide your condition, and then having to struggle on when symptoms are at their peak, does no one any favours. Be open and honest about it. Explain that there will be some days in the summer when you are incapable of total commitment and concentration. More people will then understand when you are in difficulty and will not simply think you are swinging the lead and looking for an excuse to have some time off.

Chapter 3
Why Do People Get
Asthma and Hay Fever?

Asthma and hay fever are both related to the respiratory system. Asthma affects the lungs and hay fever affects the nose and the throat – though other parts of the body, including the eyes and the skin, can also be involved. But there is more to it than this simple fact.

The basic link is allergy. Both conditions are mostly caused because the sufferer's body reacts violently to some substance breathed in, eaten or touched. It is this allergy that brings about the changes in the breathing system that lead to the symptoms of hay fever or asthma.

And there is also another link. One in every three people who have asthma also suffer from hay fever. Clearly, their bodies are unusually sensitive.

What is an allergy?

To truly understand, you need to remember that all living species have but one basic aim – survival! Without reproduction, no species can survive; and many things can affect the ability to reproduce. A species can be hunted by other animals, for instance; or it can be wiped out completely by disease.

Elephants, for example, now face extinction because they have been hunted by humans for so long that the numbers left to reproduce have dwindled. But before humans came on the scene and slaughtered them, elephants were faced with different threats – they were hunted down by other animals. So elephants developed ways of surviving. They gathered together in herds to put off predators. That also meant that they remained in close proximity to each other, increasing their reproductive capacity. They also developed loud trumpeting noises to frighten predators and warn other elephants of danger. Those were both attempts to keep the species alive.

Humans have developed similar methods to rid themselves of threats to the survival of their own species. But humans are no longer hunted by other animals. Their biggest threat comes from small things, like microbes, that cause disease. But unlike elephants, they often can't even see the things that are dangerous.

Happily, human beings and other animals have developed an internal mechanism to deal with such threats. It is called the immune system; and it is ever-watchful to handle those threats to survival that are so tiny that they cannot be seen.

It is this immune system that presents the problem for people with asthma and hay fever. For some reason, their inner defence mechanisms interpret things as a threat to their survival, when in fact they are not. There is a mix-up that makes their immune systems think that something breathed in, eaten or touched, is dangerous.

In other words, the internal defence mechanism designed to help to ensure survival has actually become the problem. The immune system lets them down and they become "allergic" to substances that the bodies of normal people do not see as threatening.

That, in essence, is an allergy. It is the immune system's response to an event that is not really a danger at all. The body's defence system has become confused – it sees something as highly dangerous when, in fact, it is quite harmless.

What is the immune system?

The immune system is a complicated mechanism that provides a belt and braces approach to protecting us from invisible invaders. It is the internal equivalent of the elephant's trumpeting.

White blood cells form the key part of the immune system. These can ward off potentially harmful invaders in a number of different ways. When something enters the body through the skin, nose or mouth, it inevitably ends up in the bloodstream. There, the white cells should be able to deal with the (harmful) invader. One way is for the cell to swallow the particle whole – sealing it inside itself, never again to see the light of day. Another approach is for the white blood cell to produce a special chemical, known as an antibody, on its surface. When the invading substance comes into contact with this antibody, it sticks firmly to it and is so rendered harmless.

But the defence mechanism of the immune system doesn't end there.

Although invaders are made harmless by the antibodies, the immune system likes to make sure. So, as soon as something gets stuck onto an antibody, other chemicals are produced by the body to go out on the attack. A substance called histamine is made by the cells next to our blood vessels. The main job of this chemical is to increase the power of the antibodies to enable the body to get rid of the offending item more quickly. However, like many other chemicals, histamine causes side effects – swelling and inflammation, which are the leading symptoms of hay fever and asthma.

People with asthma and hay fever produce an abnormally high quantity of one particular kind of antibody. Because there is such a large supply of this antibody, a great deal of histamine is released. That leads to the inflammation and swelling that signals the beginning of an attack. In people with normal levels of antibodies, the smaller amount of histamine released doesn't cause a problem.

What are antigens?

An antigen is any substance capable of being stuck to an antibody. In serious disease, it may be a chemical on the surface of a bacteria.

For instance, most people in the UK have been vaccinated against tuberculosis. This vaccine, which most people receive during their teens, leads the body to produce an antibody. If the person then becomes infected with the tuberculosis bacteria, a chemical on the surface of the bug is attracted to the antibody. The result is that the bug is rendered harmless – it is stuck to the antibody where it eventually dies. The threat to the survival of the individual exposed to tuberculosis is ended, thanks to the antibody.

Similarly, when you suffer from some childhood disease, like chickenpox, your body is stimulated to produce antibodies. Once these are established in your bloodstream, they fight off the invading virus. Thankfully, these antibodies remain in your system forever. So if you ever meet the chickenpox virus again, your body will fight it off before you can suffer any symptoms.

However, viruses and bacteria are not the only antigens that can stick to antibodies in your bloodstream. Any chemical or particle can, potentially, become an antigen. The antigens of people with asthma and hay fever are any of a wide variety of substances that can stick to the particular antibody of which they have an excess.

The antigens that can trigger either of these conditions vary immensely. Something that leads to hay fever in one individual may cause no trouble in another. Similarly, something that causes an asthma attack in one child, may pass another by. However, there are two very common antigens that very often do cause trouble. These are pollen and the droppings of the house dust mite.

Pollens from grass and trees are the most common antigens for hay fever. Pollens are one half of the reproductive system of many plants – they are released by the plant and float through the air in the hope that they meet another plant and reproduce.

The droppings of the house dust mite are the most common antigens leading to asthma. House dust mites are tiny creatures that feed on house dust, particularly on the tiny particles of skin that we shed each day. They are to be found in every house and are most common in temperate, relatively humid climates – as in the UK!

Between them, house dust mites and pollen are responsible for about 80% of all cases of asthma and hay fever.

Food allergies

Even though air-born allergens are responsible for the vast majority of cases of asthma and hay fever, others suffer because they are allergic to certain foods.

Food allergies were once dismissed by the medical profession; but there is now widespread acceptance that many individuals are allergic to certain foodstuffs and to the chemicals used in food production. It appears that our digestive system hasn't adapted sufficiently to cope with modern diets. Our bodies require a much more varied diet than they now receive; and they also sometimes cannot tolerate the additives and the chemicals that we eat constantly.

Food allergy is not such a strange concept. We all probably know of someone who has a violent reaction to shellfish. This commonly produces a rapid flushing of the face in people who are allergic to it. They also can swell up and panic as a result of the shellfish affecting their breathing. After this reaction has happened for the first time, they realise that they can never eat shellfish again and they avoid it religiously.

Food may be causing the problem for people with asthma. Consequently, the possibility of a food allergy should really be considered by people with this condition.

Histamine

No sooner does someone with excess antibodies come into contact with an allergen, such as food, dust mite droppings, or a pollen, the offending substance attaches to the antibodies and histamine is released. Because the victim has large numbers of antibodies, a large number of antigens can become attached. That leads to the release of significant amounts of histamine – in turn producing the symptoms of hay fever and asthma. It is the ability of histamine to cause swelling and inflammation that produces the symptoms.

In the nose, for example, excess histamine causes swelling and inflammation of the nasal passages. This makes the nose run, and the tubes become narrower than normal. The victim feels bunged up and stuffy. Sneezing might also begin in an attempt to clear the nose. The result of excess histamine is a stuffy nose, a runny nose and sneezing – the typical reactions of someone with hay fever.

Histamine behaves differently in the lungs. It inflames the tubes of the airways, causing them to produce liquid (phlegm). The result is that the tubes become narrower, making breathing more difficult. That leads to the wheezing and the attempts to draw deep breaths that are clear signs of asthma.

Because asthma and hay fever are dependent upon one particular kind of antibody being produced in excess, many people are susceptible to both conditions. One day the antigen may be the droppings of the house dust mite, leading to an asthma attack. On another day, tree pollen may produce a bout of hay fever.

Overreaction

The problem for people with asthma and hay fever is that their body has overreacted to the apparent threat of house dust mites, foodstuffs and pollens.

Clearly, it is very unlikely, for example, that the droppings of house dust mites will endanger the survival of the human species. For tuberculosis though, the threat is real; and the population would be at risk if we did not have antibodies to the tuberculosis bug. That's what happened with bubonic plague in London, for instance; and that's why the World Health Organisation is so keen to find a vaccine for AIDS. There is a real threat to human life in the Third World because we have no effective antibodies to counter the virus.

But the droppings of house dust mites, or the pollen from the grass on your lawn, are hardly the same as the virus that leads to AIDS or bubonic plague! However, people with asthma and hay fever have an immune system that seems to think these harmless substances are equally danger-ous. Their immune systems have overreacted; and they suffer the symptoms we call hay fever or asthma as the result.

Quite why some people should be born with this in-built overreaction remains a mystery. We do know that the tendency to have excess, overre-acting antibodies runs in families – and that points to a genetic cause. It may well be that there is some kind of genetic malfunction that causes people to develop this kind of overreaction.

However, not all sufferers are born with this problem; some develop hay fever or asthma in later life. For some reason, their immune system suddenly starts to manufacture the excess antibodies – something unknown triggers off an increase in antibody production in individuals not genetically pre-disposed to the condition.

This question has been puzzling doctors in recent years. Why is it that asthma and hay fever appears to run in families, presumably with a genetic link, yet some people develop these conditions in later life with no evidence of a previous family history of the ailments? Why is it that some cases of hay fever and asthma appear to pop up with no easily identifiable genetic link? Why is it that some people suddenly start to produce antibod-ies to harmless substances like house dust mite droppings or pollen? Why should a normal human immune system suddenly perceive pollen, for instance, as a threat?

Pollution

Some doctors and researchers are coming to the conclusion that pollution is the missing link – for asthma in particular, but also for hay fever.

There is growing evidence that pollution makes people, who would not otherwise suffer from these conditions, become sensitised to the allergens that trigger attacks. In other words, it may be that pollution is turning more and more people into asthma or hay fever sufferers.

Figures on hay fever emphasise the potential effect of pollution. Hay fever is four times as common as it was 20 years ago – yet the level of pollen in the atmosphere has fallen! Something else must be causing more and more people to become hypersensitive. Experts increasingly blame pollution.

Research in America, the UK, Finland and Germany has pointed specifically to traffic pollution. It has been clearly demonstrated at St Bartholomew's Hospital, London, that specific pollutants such as fumes from cars and lorries can trigger asthma attacks.

Investigators also believe that pollution can make otherwise normal people more likely to suffer from asthma and hay fever. This means that pollution may be the answer to the question why non-genetically-disposed individuals suddenly become victims of asthma or hay fever. Fumes from cars and lorries may be causing their bodies to become hypersensitive to allergens.

Some scientists, politicians and civil servants say this is all very well but there is no proof. More work is needed, they insist. But doctors in London's hospitals can predict when their wards will fill with asthma patients – they simply look out of the window first thing in the morning. If the air is smoggy and polluted, they know their wards will fill up as the morning develops. Proof it may not be; but to people with asthma there is no doubt that pollution certainly makes their condition worse.

Is the immune system always to blame?

For most people, the immune system is involved in some way with asthma or hay fever.

Pollen or house dust mite droppings may not always trigger it into producing histamine – though they are the most common causes. Cat fur can also produce asthma, as can certain foods to which individuals are allergic – particularly dyes and preservatives used in manufactured food-stuffs. Similarly, some people get hay fever from contact with feathers or hair.

What all these triggers have in common is their ability to produce histamine as a result of an antibody reaction. All of them cause an allergic reaction involving the immune system. For the vast majority of asthma sufferers and for all hay fever sufferers, an allergy of one kind or another is at the root of their trouble.

Nevertheless, a proportion of asthma victims do not have any obvious allergy, yet still suffer from the condition. These people have particularly sensitive lungs – as do all asthma sufferers. But unlike the majority of asthmatics, whose lungs react after contact with an allergen, these non-allergy sufferers have lungs that are so sensitive that they can become inflamed and phlegmy from the simplest cause.

Cold air is one example of a cause of asthma in non-allergy patients. Exercise too can also lead to attacks of asthma in people whose lungs are sensitive. Even stress has been shown to play a major role in the likelihood of asthma attacks in people whose lungs are hypersensitive.

So, although the immune system is often to blame for asthma, some people suffer because their lungs are over-sensitive, or as doctors say hyperreactive. For people with hay fever, the immune system is always involved.

The final analysis

The answer to the question "Why do people get asthma or hay fever?" is relatively straightforward. All our bodies are designed to ward off potential threats to our survival. But for sufferers, their immune systems have become overactive – geared up to protect their bodies from things that are not real threats; or else their lungs have become over-sensitive to normal stimulants like cold air.

All in all, people with asthma or hay fever have biological response mechanisms that are much more highly developed than in so-called normal people. The penalty is that such highly geared systems bring large amounts of histamine in their wake; and that is where the problems begin.

But whatever the cause of an individual's symptoms, it is vital that the problem is attended to properly and promptly. Asthma is a serious disease and it can kill. Only by treating it as a real problem can the number of deaths be reduced.

Chapter 4
Medical Treatment for Asthma

Bronchodilators

The mainstay of medical treatment of asthma is a group of drugs with the power to open up the patient's airways. Such drugs are called bronchodilators because they dilate, or open up, the bronchial tubes to enable the patient to breathe more easily. Virtually every asthma patient is given bronchodilator treatment. The most popular bronchodilators are drugs like salbutamol (sold as VENTOLIN), which are most frequently taken using a special device called an inhaler.

How do bronchodilators work?

Most bronchodilators work by stimulating a particular cell into action. When this happens, one of the main effects is the inhibition of the release of histamine – which leads to a reduction in inflammation and fluid release.

Bronchodilators have other effects. They also help to relax the smooth muscles of the airways (tubes in the lungs), which allows them to widen. These drugs also stop the release of chemicals within the lungs that can contribute to an asthma attack.

Because of the way they work, bronchodilators are particularly useful in the treatment of episodes of wheeziness. When someone with asthma feels tightness in the chest and hears the breathing becoming more wheezy, a quick dose of bronchodilator immediately reduces the symptoms.

There is also a good deal of evidence that, because bronchodilators open up the airways, they are also useful in preventing attacks of asthma and episodes of wheeziness. For this reason, doctors usually prescribe bronchodilators for everyday use – rather than just for during an attack.

Taking the main kinds of bronchodilators

Most asthma patients take these bronchodilators by means of an inhaler. There are various kinds of inhalers on the market; but they all work in basically the same way. The drug is breathed in. This brings small particles of the drug directly into contact with the area in which it is needed – the inside of the lungs.

Inhaling bronchodilators has an important further benefit. Breathing in the drug prevents it from reaching parts of the body other than the lungs. If the bronchodilator is swallowed or injected, the drug is then also absorbed by other organs and tissues – with a risk of side effects. A lesser amount is available for the lungs; and doctors need to prescribe higher doses to make up for this loss – again with increased risk of side effects.

When the drug is given in tablet form, it takes far longer to get round the body and reach the lungs. Relief of symptoms is therefore much slower if bronchodilators are given in this way.

Tablets and injections of bronchodilators are occasionally necessary for young children who cannot cope with an inhaler, and when a victim has collapsed during an attack.

On the whole, though, doctors prefer patients to use an inhaler whenever possible. The bronchodilator reaches the lungs quickly, doses can be kept lower and the level of side effects is minimal.

Inhalers

Inhalers come in a variety of shapes and sizes.

Puffers

The most popular inhaler is a pressurised aerosol, commonly called a puffer. It works much like a hair spray.

The drug, in liquid form, is forced into the small can under pressure. When the top of the can is pressed, the drug is released through the mouthpiece. It comes out very quickly, still as a liquid. But the small liquid droplets evaporate rapidly, leaving minute particles to be breathed in.

The amount of drug released when you press the top of the canister is precisely measured by the inhaler itself. You will therefore sometimes hear doctors call them metered-dose inhalers – because they measure the amount of drug you are taking.

Autohalers

Another kind of inhaler, the Autohaler, delivers a specified amount of drug. But you do not need to press the top of the can as you would for a puffer. You simply breathe in while holding the device to your mouth; and this sucking action automatically releases the drug.

Rotahalers and Spinhalers

A Rotahaler uses capsules of powdered drug instead of a liquid. The capsule is placed inside the device, where it is broken open. When you breathe in, a fan inside the inhaler whirls around and blows the tiny particles of powder into your mouth.

Another device called a Spinhaler works on similar principles.

Turbohalers

The Turbohaler also uses powdered drugs; but, unlike the Rotahaler, it is capable of delivering more than one dose. A Turbohaler has enough drug inside it for 100 doses; but only delivers the amount of powder necessary for each inhalation.

As such, the Turbohaler is much like the puffer – except that puffers use liquid drugs and usually contain more doses within the canister.

Diskhalers

The Diskhaler is flat and wide in comparison to the other inhalers, which are tube-like. A circular disk, containing eight doses of bronchodilator, is placed inside it.

To use a Diskhaler, you lift up the lid before breathing in. This turns the disk to move a new dose to the right position and then punctures the foil surrounding the drug. The powder is released when you breathe in – very much as in other dry-powder inhalers.

On the whole, doctors prefer to prescribe puffers that use liquid drugs. This is the most effective way of getting the right amount of drug to your lungs as quickly as possible.

However, using a puffer requires a bit of skill; and the other kinds of inhalers that contain dry powder are a bit easier to operate. So these are often reserved for patients who find it difficult to use a puffer.

Using an inhaler

One of the biggest problems with asthma care is caused by incorrect use of inhalers. Studies have shown that many asthma attacks are due to the fact that patients are not getting the right dose of drugs as a result of using their inhalers improperly.

That's not necessarily the fault of asthma sufferers, for other studies have shown that not all family doctors are well versed in the use of these devices either! So, if someone who doesn't have asthma and doesn't really know exactly how to use an inhaler tries to explain what to do to an anxious patient, the result is not always ideal.

Fortunately, things are now improving. Most family doctors get their practice nurses, specially trained in using inhalers, to describe the technique to asthma patients. Research suggests that patients are less anxious when discussing things with a nurse than they are with a doctor, and are thus more likely to remember what they were told. So, if your GP explains how to use the inhaler and you are not quite sure about it, ask the practice nurse to go over it again. Your treatment is going to be much more effective if you get the inhaler technique right.

Metered-dose aerosol inhalers that use liquid drugs (puffers), do need a little co-ordination to use properly. The correct way to use an inhaler is as follows:

1 Remove the cover from the mouthpiece.
2 Shake the device up and down quite sharply.
3 Breathe out gently, but not completely.
4 Pop the mouthpiece of the inhaler into your mouth and close your lips around it.
5 Breathe in slowly.
6 Just after you have started to breathe in, press the top of the aerosol can.
7 Hold your breath for about ten seconds after breathing in.
8 Carry on breathing normally.

The usual dose for most people with asthma is two puffs – so you need to repeat the process about 30 seconds later. However, each asthma patient will have an individual treatment plan, so never change your dose unless your doctor has told you to do so.

The problems with inhaler technique are two-fold. First, it is sometimes difficult for people to get the hang of pressing the top of the aerosol just after they have started to breathe in. Second, people sometimes do not hold their breath for long enough.

Both faults cause you to get less drug than you need to control your condition. If you do not start breathing in first before pressing the canister, you run the risk of the drug sticking inside your mouth when it squirts out of the aerosol; by breathing in first you automatically suck the drug in to your lungs. If you do not hold your breath for at least ten seconds, the drug doesn't have enough time to get deep down inside the lungs; by breathing out too quickly you expel some of the drug, so not enough gets to work in treating the asthma.

If you just can't get the knack of using an inhaler, go back to see the practice nurse for extra tuition. Do try to get on with the aerosol inhalers, for they offer the best range of benefits of treatment.

If you just can't cope, your doctor may decide to change your treatment to a dry-powder inhaler which does not require you to press the canister – the drug is delivered automatically as you breathe in. With a dry-powder inhaler you only have one action to worry about – so using it is much easier. The doctor may also suggest a spacer device.

Spacer devices

Spacer devices are extension tubes that are added to the mouthpiece of the inhaler. With a spacer, you do not need to get your timing absolutely right; and you no longer have to be sure that you start breathing in first before pressing the aerosol.

Some people also prefer to use a spacer device because they find the sudden jet of aerosol uncomfortable when it first rushes into their mouth. However, a spacer is bulky and less convenient to carry than the inhaler on its own.

Other ways of taking bronchodilators

Syrups are available as well as tablets and injections. These are mostly used for babies and very young children who cannot cope with inhalers.

For people with severe asthma, a nebuliser may be required.

Nebulisers

A nebuliser makes a fine mist out of a liquid by blowing oxygen through it.

There are various kinds of nebuliser. In hospitals they tend to be large devices attached to oxygen cylinders; but a portable machine with a small air pump is more usual in the home. There is also a nebuliser machine that creates a mist, without pumping air through it, by the use of rapid vibration to break up the bronchodilator liquid.

Nebulisers are usually used for patients with severe chronic asthma, who cannot rely on inhalers alone and for children and babies who cannot use an inhaler.

Nebulisers are also employed for the relief of acute attacks of asthma – GPs usually carry a nebuliser in the car to treat emergencies.

Using a nebuliser is straightforward. You first place a dose of the drug in the special chamber of the machine. Then you switch on the machine, place the mask over your nose and mouth, and breathe normally. Sometimes, the machine has a mouthpiece, instead of a mask, and you should breathe through this.

You can be taught how to use a nebuliser by the practice nurse. You will also be shown how to take the device to pieces and clean it thoroughly – nebulisers must be kept clean to operate efficiently. Also be sure to have the pump serviced every three months or so – without this regular check, it could fail in the middle of an attack, just when you need it most.

Other types of bronchodilators

Although the bronchodilators that act on special cells are the mainstay of asthma treatment these days, other types of bronchodilator are also in common use.

One of these is a drug that acts on the nervous system to relax the muscles of the airways and open up the tubes. It is available for use as a puffer inhaler or in a nebuliser.

Another range of bronchodilators is related to caffeine. These are not used in an inhaler or nebuliser and are mostly given by injection to patients with attacks of asthma. They are also available in tablet form and in syrups.

Steroid treatment of asthma

Bronchodilators are effective in relieving asthma symptoms and also in helping to reduce the likelihood of attacks. Their effect is instantaneous and can be very powerful – such as, for example, in the case of an injection of theophylline.

However, more needs to be done for a large number of patients than is possible with bronchodilators alone. For this reason, steroid treatment is also prescribed for many patients with asthma.

There are many myths about steroids; and one of the reasons why some asthma patients do not have their condition properly controlled is because they refuse to take their drugs once they know they are steroids.

One asthma specialist did some research with patients with serious asthma that could not be treated effectively. He found that the patients, all children, were not taking the drugs prescribed by their GPs. Their parents had realised that the medicines were steroids and so stopped their children from taking the full dosage prescribed. As soon as the specialist ensured that these children received the proper doses of the steroids, their asthma came under control.

Parents who forbid their youngsters steroid therapy, or reduce the dose for fear of side effects, are actually taking high risks – even of death in bad cases. There is abundant evidence that steroids are very effective in treating asthma; and so to avoid this therapy on the basis of ill-informed speculation about the effects of these drugs is foolish as well as dangerous.

People are often worried by the word steroid. It is not a code name for a nasty or evil substance, but is just a name given to a certain type of chemical structure – a steroid chemical is one that has a specific group of atoms in a particular arrangement. This means that there are many different types of steroids.

There is one type that can increase your muscle power. These drugs are banned for use by international athletes. They are the type of steroid that most people worry about – potentially dangerous and with nasty side effects, including fatality.

But there are other steroids. For example the contraceptive pill, one of the safest pharmaceutical products known, is a steroid. So too are the chemicals produced in the liver that help break down the fat we eat. And cholesterol – vital for life (though not in excess!) is also a steroid.

The steroids used to treat asthma are not like those used by unscrupulous athletes – the danger steroids. Those prescribed for asthma are the same as the ones produced by the adrenal gland – the small gland that sits on top of each kidney and releases hormones such as adrenaline. These steroids help asthmatics by slowly reducing the amount of inflammation and swelling in the airways. They also diminish the amount of phlegm secreted by the lungs. But, unlike bronchodilators, their effect is gradual – so steroids are not useful for inhalation during wheezy episodes.

Using steroids

Most people who are prescribed steroids, such as beclomethasone (sold as BECOTIDE) will use them in puffers or other kinds of inhalers. They are taken regularly and not just when the patient feels wheezy.

Most people take their steroids twice a day. It takes about two weeks for them to begin to have their effect. This causes a problem, for some people give up steroid therapy too soon. They think after a few days that the drug is not working; and fail to realise that they need to wait for at least a fortnight before telling whether or not it is effective.

Another reason for the apparent failure of steroid therapy is that asthma sufferers stop using the inhaler as soon as they feel better. It's precisely because of the steroids that they do feel so well. So, never give up steroid treatment without first discussing things with your doctor. To do so could expose you to the risk of a severe attack.

Steroid therapy for asthma is noticeably difficult because of the myths about these drugs and their side-effects. Many of those who do not comply fully with the doctor's instructions – they stop taking them as soon as they feel well again, or they take less than the prescribed dose – are not getting their condition treated adequately. Their lungs are allowed to become inflamed unnecessarily.

Side-effects from inhaled steroids are very unlikely. The treatment, in small doses, goes straight to where it is needed and very little is absorbed by other tissues and organs. The most common steroid-related side effect is an increased incidence of mouth and gum infections; but these disappear if the patient uses a mouthwash after inhaling.

Steroid treatment of asthma is a long-term therapy to reduce inflammation of the airways, and is not suitable for dealing with attacks of wheezing. For this reason, many patients on steroids will also need a bronchodilator. They take their two steroid doses each day and then top up with puffs of bronchodilator when needed. In essence, steroid treatment of asthma is a preventative therapy.

Other preventative treatments

Steroids are just one of the groups of drugs that doctors prescribe for the prevention of asthma attacks. However, because allergy is behind most cases of asthma, anti-allergy drugs have also proved useful.

Sodium cromoglycate (sold as INTAL) is the anti-allergy drug most widely used. Although it was introduced 30 years ago, scientists are still not sure precisely how it produces its effect. What is known is that it interferes with the chemical processes in the airways that cause the release of chemicals to make the muscles contract. Bronchodilators work by ensuring that the airways open up; and cromoglycate works by preventing the closure of the airways from happening in the first place.

INTAL is taken in an inhaler, usually four times a day, as preventative medication. It has no effect on episodes of wheeziness – but it can prevent allergic reactions. For instance, if asthma is worsened by contact with animal fur, taking sodium cromoglycate before coming into contact with a pet will prevent wheeziness from occurring.

Sodium cromoglycate and drugs like it appear to be most effective in children.

It also seems that the required dosage of steroids and some bronchodilators can be reduced by the use of preventative treatment of this kind.

This means that some asthma sufferers may face the prospect of having three different types of inhaler – a preventative inhaler to stop the allergic reaction, a steroid inhaler to provide long term bronchodilation, and an inhaler that contains a bronchodilator to treat episodes of wheeziness and chest tightness.

Adverse reactions

The main worry about taking any medicine is its potential side effects. Indeed, one of the reasons why steroids are not taken properly by many people with asthma is the fear of side effects.

It's worth pausing to think about what doctors mean by side effects. They mean anything, literally anything, that is not the main effect of the drug. Hence side effects are not necessarily bad. For example, the oral contraceptive pill is designed to stop women from becoming pregnant; but one of its side effects is to prevent ovarian cancer. Now most people would see that as a benefit and not describe it as a side effect – yet doctors would so describe it because it is not the main purpose of the preparation.

This definition is important because it is a legal requirement to provide information about side effects on the packaging of pharmaceuticals. The long list in small print on the package makes it seem as though the drug you are about to take has many harmful actions. That's because the public understanding of a side effect is not the same as the medical definition.

You may find beneficial side effects, in addition to the main therapeutic action, in the small-print list. That's why it is preferable to talk about adverse reactions rather than side effects. These are the reactions you might have to the drug which are unpleasant and harmful.

Adverse reactions to the bronchodilators vary according to the exact one prescribed. However, because inhaled bronchodilators go directly to where they are needed, adverse reactions are rarely seen. Of course, for inhaled bronchodilators, the drug does come into contact with the mouth; and so this is the place where trouble can occur. The most likely adverse reaction there is a feeling of sheer unpleasantness caused by the rush of the drug into the mouth. That can largely be overcome by using a spacer device.

Adverse reactions are more likely if the drug is not inhaled, but taken by injection or as a tablet or syrup. The medication then comes into contact with parts of the body other than the lungs. It is also far more difficult to get the dosage right.

In these instances, bronchodilators can cause a mild shaking of the hands. Increases in heart rate have also been experienced, as have the occurrence of occasional headaches and stomach upsets. Sometimes injections can cause pain where the needle is inserted. In all these instances, the adverse reactions are dose-related. That means that the reaction lessens as the dose is reduced; and it worsens as the dose is increased. There have been no reports of irreversible adverse reactions to bronchodilators.

The incidence of adverse reactions to steroids is very low indeed, providing the drugs are inhaled. Mouth irritations can occur, but these can be avoided with proper oral hygiene. However, the incidence of adverse reactions rises when steroids are taken in tablet form or by injection.

The main problem is in children, whose growth can become retarded and faces bloated as a result of high doses. As a result, doctors are very careful indeed about steroids that are not inhaled; and any doses given in tablet form will be very low and will be monitored carefully by special clinics.

Sodium cromoglycate can sometimes cause coughing, especially when inhaled in the powder form. The powder can also irritate the throat.

Taken as a whole, adverse reactions to modern asthma medicines are rare. Considering that nearly three million people take puffs of drugs every day, and that this has been happening for 30 years or so, it is a remarkable achievement to have produced modern therapies that are so trouble free.

But that doesn't mean you can relax entirely! Adverse reactions should always be reported to your GP as soon as possible. And you can avoid many reactions by taking the drugs exactly as prescribed, by getting reliable tuition from practice nurses, by keeping the inhaler mouthpiece clean and by rinsing your mouth with water after each inhalation.

Summary

No complete cure for asthma has yet been discovered. The principal aim of treatment is to reduce the inflammation, often by the inhibition in one way or another of the effects of allergens. This may be done by avoiding the allergen altogether – as in removing certain foods from the diet – or it may mean drug control, or both.

However, like all drugs, medicines for asthma do have potential adverse reactions. These are most easily avoided if the drug can be delivered directly to its site of action – the lungs. By delivering the drug in this way, other parts of the body are not so easily exposed to the drug's action, minimising the problems and increasing the amount of drug available to the problem area.

Steroids are very useful; and many people would be far better treated if they did not continue to believe that steroids are inherently harmful. When used properly, they have a great deal to offer.

Chapter 5
Medical Treatment for Hay Fever

There is as yet no complete cure for hay fever. Medical treatment is focused on combating the same chemical that causes the trouble in asthma – histamine.

Antihistamines are the principal drugs used to reduce the symptoms of hay fever. They are very effective for hay fever, but are of little use in asthma treatment as they have no effect on problems such as the narrowing of the airways by muscular contraction.

Antihistamines

A wide variety of antihistamines is available, either in tablet or in syrup form. A few may be given by injection.

Some antihistamines can only be obtained by prescription from your doctor. Others are available without prescription, but only from a chemist. You cannot buy antihistamines from a supermarket or from a non-pharmacy drug store.

Antihistamines are very effective because they stop the histamine from having its inflammatory effect – the nose doesn't run and the throat doesn't become irritated.

However, antihistamines for hay fever also have their problems. Because they only work as tablets or syrups or injections, the whole of your body is exposed to them. This causes the cells that release histamine throughout the body to become blocked by the drug – even in areas where histamine is not causing a problem. There is more likelihood of adverse reactions in these circumstances, as compared to a situation in which the drug is delivered directly to where it is needed – as in the case of nasal sprays.

Adverse reactions

Adverse reactions with antihistamines are much more common than with asthma preparations, even though they are safe enough to buy over the counter without a prescription.

The most common problem is drowsiness. You will often see a warning on the packet, advising you not to drive or operate machinery while taking the drug. You should not drink alcohol either, for the combination will make you very drowsy indeed. There are newer antihistamine preparations which do not cause drowsiness – but there are fewer of them on the market and only one is available without prescription.

Whatever the antihistamine, adverse reactions can include headaches, a dry mouth and a reduction in the number of times urine is passed. Also, antihistamines cause particular problems for people with epilepsy, liver disease and glaucoma. So although antihistamines can deal very effectively with hay fever, they are not without their difficulties.

Doctors suggest therefore that the patient should start off with a less complicated remedy. If that works, he or she will not need to be troubled by the complications of antihistamines, even though they remain the main-stay of hay fever treatment.

Decongestants

Decongestants should always be tried first to counter the symptoms of hay fever. Although these can be taken as tablets, they are far better delivered by nasal spray directly to where they are needed. Nasal sprays and eye drops are used to stem the flow of the fluids and stop the nose from running and the eyes from watering.

Decongestants work by constricting the blood vessels in the nose or around the eyes. This reduces the swelling and so lessens the irritation, resulting in a smaller amount of fluid release from the affected area.

When using a nasal spray, it is best to bend backward so that the droplets go up the nose and don't run out again. To use a nasal spray properly do it as follows:

1 Lie down on the bed with the top of your head over the edge, pointing towards the floor (this way you should be looking up to the ceiling).
2 Blow your nose gently to clear the nostrils.
3 Shake the container up and down.
4 Place your finger on one nostril to close it.
5 Insert the container into the other nostril.
6 Gently breathe in.
7 Press the container to emit a puff of spray just after you start to breathe in.

8 Breathe out through your mouth.
9 Repeat the procedure for the other nostril.
10 Wipe the nosepiece of the spray with tissue.

Most decongestants are available over the counter. Some are not available on the NHS. Your doctor can prescribe them; but you have to pay the full cost of a private prescription.

If you use decongestants too frequently, their effect will reduce as your system gets accustomed to them. So take decongestants wisely. Reserve them for when symptoms are at their worst rather than using them steadily throughout the hay fever season.

Steroids

Steroids are very useful indeed for people with hay fever.

There are many myths about steroids; and one of the reasons why some patients do not have their condition properly controlled is because they refuse to take their drugs once they know they are steroids. (The following paragraphs on steroids are repeated from Chapter 4 for the benefit of hay fever sufferers who may not have read the section on steroids and asthma).

People are often worried by the word steroid. It is not a code name for a nasty or evil substance, but is just a name given to a certain type of chemical structure – a steroid chemical is one that has a specific group of atoms in a particular arrangement. This means that there are many different types of steroids.

There is one type that can increase your muscle power. These drugs are banned for use by international athletes. They are the type of steroid that most people worry about – potentially dangerous and with nasty side effects, including fatality.

But there are other steroids. For example the contraceptive pill, one of the safest pharmaceutical products known, is a steroid. So too are the chemicals produced in the liver that help break down the fat we eat. And cholesterol – vital for life (though not in excess!) is also a steroid.

The steroids used to treat hay fever are not like those used by unscrupulous athletes – the danger steroids. Those prescribed for hay fever are the same as the ones produced by the adrenal gland – the small gland that sits on top of each kidney and releases hormones such as adrenaline. These steroids help people with hay fever because they slowly reduce the amount of inflammation and swelling. These drugs also diminish the amount of fluid secreted by the nasal passages.

Nasal sprays of steroids are particularly effective against hay fever that does not respond to decongestants or antihistamines. One of the most popular of these nasal sprays, BECONASE, is now available over the counter.

To use nasal spray steroids, follow the instructions on using such sprays in the above section on decongestants.

Steroids in low doses may sometimes be given as tablets; but usually only for patients who require short-term relief that cannot be achieved in any other way.

Other hay fever drugs

A range of anti-allergy drugs can also be taken for hay fever. Drugs used for asthma, such as sodium cromoglycate, work by interfering with the release of histamine – see Chapter 4.

But most people find that their hay fever can be controlled adequately by decongestants or over-the-counter antihistamines.

Food avoidance

One of the other methods of controlling hay fever symptoms is food avoidance. Food allergies, particularly troublesome for people with asthma, also play a role in the severity of hay fever symptoms. Therefore, doctors will often suggest that food allergies are tested for and appropriate action taken.

The best way of avoiding symptoms due to food allergies is to stop eating the foodstuff responsible. You may need to talk to a dietician about this; and the practice nurse at your local GP's surgery can help as well. Also, look at the section on exclusion diets in Chapter 1.

E numbers

Some food additives, often referred to by their E numbers, may cause problems and should be avoided whenever possible.

The most troublesome E numbers are those in the range 220 to 227. These are preservatives that contain chemicals called sulphites. Sulphites release sulphur dioxide into the air; and it is sulphur dioxide, also present in air pollution, that appears to be responsible for triggering attacks of hay fever and asthma in susceptible people.

You may well find that you will suffer from symptoms after taking food containing the sulphite-based preservatives commonly used in sausages, pre-washed salads and fizzy drinks. The answer is to read the labels carefully and avoid anything that contains E220 to E227.

Medical treatment of hay fever

Most people rely on preparations they can buy over the counter in a chemist's shop rather than trouble their doctor with what they think is a relatively minor complaint. They do not realise that the doctor has far more powerful treatments at his or her disposal than the pharmacist. And so they continue to suffer from irritating symptoms.

Yet hay fever can be quite serious, severely limiting work and social life. It can even be totally disabling for short periods. So a visit to the doctor to get an effective treatment is important for most sufferers from hay fever.

Chapter 6
Alternative Therapy

It's always worthwhile remembering that many therapies once thought of as "alternative" treatments are now accepted as orthodox medicine.

For instance, osteopathy, which treats problems like back pain, was once considered as alternative, with many doctors dismissing its practice as hocus pocus. Now it's available on the NHS. Similarly, acupuncture, once thought by many doctors to be a strange and unwarranted practice of eastern mystics, is now on offer at many pain clinics in general hospitals; and some anaesthetists learn it as part of their training. Years ago, modern drugs were viewed with suspicion; now it is often difficult to leave the GP's surgery without a prescription.

Orthodox medicine tends to dismiss things it hasn't invented as alternative, untried or even dangerous. What orthodox medicine is reluctant to admit is that most people who visit a GP will get better no matter what the doctor does. In other words, there is an awful lot of hocus pocus in orthodox medicine.

Modern medicine can and has performed miracles in some cases; but many of the most important diseases have not been eradicated by medicine alone but also by improvements in standards of hygiene and the supply of uncontaminated water.

The result of all this is that if you suggest alternative methods of treatment for asthma, your GP will almost certainly warn you against them. You will be told that you would be placing yourself in danger of having a potentially fatal asthma attack if you decide to give up the drugs and opt for alternative treatment. You will be warned about the dangers and probably advised that some alternative therapies are harmful and that their practitioners are quacks, not properly qualified.

Your doctor probably won't lay it on so thickly if you have hay fever. You may be told to "Have a go, but don't blame me if it doesn't work".

Asthma, though, gets much more serious consideration from orthodox medical practitioners. The reason is that asthma is a very serious disease that kills 2,000 people every year. Doctors know that many asthma deaths can be prevented with the drugs at their disposal. They therefore believe that they, and they only have the answer to your disease; and that you would be foolish to try anything which is relatively untested. So, if you want to try alternative therapies, be prepared for an ear-bashing from your GP!

However, just because your GP is set against alternative remedies does not mean you should not consider them – at least as a supplement to orthodox treatment. After all, 20 years ago your GP was probably against acupuncture and now almost certainly refers patients to the local NHS pain clinic where acupuncture is available.

There is a wide range of alternative treatments available for asthma and hay fever and, providing you investigate them wisely, there is no reason why they should not be considered.

The vital thing to remember is that you should never give up your orthodox medicines without discussing the situation thoroughly with your GP or with an asthma specialist. You will be putting yourself at serious risk if your asthma is not treated effectively, however that is done.

Also, do not take up an alternative therapy without discussing it fully. You would not take an orthodox medicine like a bronchodilator without advice – so don't take up an alternative therapy without the same level of discussion.

Remember that you are dealing with your health here – and for asthma sufferers you could be dealing with your life. So be careful and consider all the options and all the advice you receive before making any changes to your treatment.

Herbalism

Herbalism is probably the oldest alternative therapy – and it is not that alternative! Many modern pharmaceuticals are made from plants and plant extracts. Aspirin for instance is based on a chemical found in a wild meadow flower and in the bark of the willow tree. Herbalism uses extracts of plants, mostly herbs. It is not as daft as some doctors would have you think.

You can buy herbal remedies at High Street chemists and in some super-markets. You can also get herbal medicines in specialist health food stores. However, you would be far better off to seek the advice of a qualified medical herbalist in the first instance. This is because, although several herbal medicines can deal with asthma and hay fever, only the herbalist is able to work out which ones are most likely to be of benefit in your particular case.

Like the doctor who has a range of bronchodilators to choose from, the herbalist has a range of plant extracts to work with. A great deal of trial and error would be involved if you were to try and decide which bronchodilator you need. Similarly, trial and error would have to govern your choice of herbal remedies. So proper advice is essential if you want to take herbal medicines for asthma or hay fever.

Medical herbalists are listed in Yellow Pages under "Herbalists". However, it is a good idea to make sure that your herbalist is a member of the National Institute of Medical Herbalists as this is an organisation that requires its members to reach particular standards of care.

Herbal remedies for asthma

Herbal remedies used in asthma can perform a number of useful functions. They can loosen the phlegm in the airways and, by making it easier to remove, effectively widen the tubes. Some herbs also have a soothing effect and reduce the irritation of the airways.

Herbs, therefore, provide symptomatic relief for asthma. They do not actually reverse an attack nor, unlike steroids, can they prevent asthma attacks from happening.

Nevertheless, many people find that herbal medicines taken regularly do help to reduce chest irritation and lessen the severity of their attacks.

Catshair

This herb, also known as asthma weed or euphorbia, can relieve the spasmodic contraction of the bronchial muscles. This spasmodic contraction of the muscles of the bronchial tubes, making it difficult to breathe, is part of the complex problem of asthma. Some herbalists also claim that the herb can prevent asthma if taken regularly.

Camomile

This is one of the most popular herbal medicines and is particularly effective in people with asthma.

According to herbalists, it can reduce the amount of spasm in the muscles of the airways and the severity of the spasmodic contraction. Camomile is also a general tonic that can make you feel more comfortable.

Horehound

This is essentially a cough remedy used in herbal cough medicines. It is useful for soothing the throat and reducing coughs, which is often a troublesome symptom for people with asthma.

Lobelia

Like catshair, according to medical herbalists this helps to reduce the spasmodic contraction of the airways.

It is also used in cough mixtures together with liquorice, which is one of the herbs reckoned to loosen phlegm inside the airways.

Nettles

Stinging nettle infusions are used to relieve episodes of wheeziness. They are also helpful in easing shortness of breath.

Herbal medicines for hay fever

Many people use herbal medicines for hay fever; and you can buy them from High Street chemist shops and drug stores. Herbal medicines are very popular for the relief of the symptoms of hay fever.

Coltsfoot

This helps relieve the throat symptoms of hay fever – the irritation in the throat and the cough that sometimes accompanies attacks. It also relieves congestion and so helps unblock a stuffy nose.

Echinacea

This is recommended as a preventative herbal medicine for hay fever. It is available in the herbal hay fever tablets called Pol'N'Count.

Garlic

This is widely recommended for hay fever. It is also available in the form of Pol'N'Count tablets.

It helps to unblock a stuffy nose and by clearing the mucus, will rid you of headaches and sneezing.

You can get garlic tablets from health food shops in a form that will prevent you from whiffing of the stuff.

Herbalists advise that, if you do eat a lot of garlic, you should chew on some parsley to neutralise the smell.

Taking herbal medicines

Your herbal remedies will be made up specifically for you if you visit a medical herbalist. Mixtures will be prepared and you may find that the herbalist concocts a special liquid made up from a selection of herbs in various measures. This is done so that the herbs attack your specific kind of symptoms.

Most herbal medicines are drunk as liquids; and you usually drink them several times each day. Your herbalist will give you specific instructions to follow.

Sometimes, you can get herbal mixtures already prepared as tablets. While these are often helpful, they may not provide the exact combination of herbs needed for your particular condition and symptoms.

Adverse reactions

Herbal medicines do not usually cause significant adverse reactions. The most common problem is that people do not like their flavour. However, high doses of lobelia-based herbal medicines can make you vomit.

Homeopathy

Compared with herbalism which is thousands of years old, homeopathy is a modern therapy. It was invented by a German doctor just over 180 years ago.

The principle behind homeopathy is that minute quantities of those substances that cause a disease can also bring about its cure.

Another basic theory is that the more dilute a medicine, the more powerful is its therapeutic potential. Orthodox medicine works in the other direction – the stronger a medicine, the greater its effect. However, this is not quite true for there is a wide range of drugs in which too high a dose has less effect than a smaller dose. Theophylline for asthma is a good example. In very high doses it causes more adverse reaction and has a reduced effect on the condition. Doctors say that drugs that work in this way have a narrow therapeutic window. In other words a lower dose is more powerful than a higher dose.

In addition to the low-dose concept of homeopathy, its practitioners also practice holistic medicine. This means that a homeopathic practitioner will treat the whole person and not just a specific symptom. Hence there is no single homeopathic medicine with which to treat asthma – but a range of possibilities. The ones chosen will depend on your individual condition, rather than just on the specific symptoms of the disease.

This approach by homeopathic medicine means that you will receive much greater benefit from the therapy if you visit a properly qualified homeopathic practitioner than if you simply buy homeopathic remedies from health food stores or High Street chemists without advice.

Of course, once the homeopath has prescribed a remedy, you will be able to get it from the High Street chemist if it is available.

Homeopaths are listed in Yellow Pages under "Homeopaths". Make sure that the practitioner you choose is a member of the Society of Homeopaths – they will have the letters RSHom after their names.

A number of orthodox medical doctors also practice homeopathy; and your own GP will be able to give you the names of local medically qualified homeopathic practitioners if you would prefer to consult one of them.

Homeopathic remedies for asthma

One approach to homeopathy for asthma is to identify the particular allergen that is causing the trouble. A suitable homeopathic medicine can then be selected; it will be a very dilute mixture of the allergen that causes the asthma attacks.

When taken, this will stimulate your system to desensitise you to the actual allergen. For instance, if you are allergic to house dust mite faeces, you can obtain a homeopathic remedy specifically targeted at reducing your sensitivity to this allergen. By taking the medicine you will stop your immune system from reacting to the dust mite droppings and hence prevent your asthma from occurring.

Another approach is to take a specific homeopathic remedy for the kind of situation in which you get asthma attacks. This emphasises the holistic approach of homeopathy. For example, if your asthma is worsened by pressure of work, the homeopath might recommend a treatment called Nux Vomica.

Almost any substance can be used in homeopathic treatment for asthma, the actual remedy prescribed depending on your specific condition.

Homeopathic remedies for hay fever

Like asthma, a homeopath will investigate the precise nature of your condition and will then prescribe the remedy most suited to your own symptoms and to the specific nature of your condition.

You will probably be prescribed a very dilute mixture of the allergen that triggers your attacks of hay fever. For example, various pollens are made into homeopathic medicines.

Using homeopathic medicines

You will be told the exact way to take your medicine according to your own individual circumstances. Most people will need to take their medicine three times a day, usually with meals.

The storage of homeopathic medicines is very important. They must be kept in the bottles provided, stored away from strong light and as far away from strong smells as possible. The bathroom cabinet, near strongly smelling soaps, is not an ideal place. Neither is your dressing table, near to perfumes or after-shaves.

Also, keep your medicines in a cool place and not near a radiator.

Adverse reactions

People may sometimes vomit when on a course of homeopathic medicines. Also skin irritation and itching can occur after taking homeopathic medicines for a while.

Homeopathic practitioners say that such symptoms show that the medicine is working as your illness is at last "coming out". However, some patients are troubled by such reactions.

Aromatherapy

Though there has been a dramatic increase in interest in aromatherapy in recent years, it is well to remember that this form of therapy was introduced in China, thousands of years ago.

The concept behind aromatherapy is that when essential oils from plants are absorbed through the skin or inhaled, they produce a range of effects – largely through the psychological reaction produced by their smell.

However, smells also have their own effect. Smelling salts, for example, were once popular to revive someone who has fainted. You can also feel physically sick after smelling a noxious substance. So aromas do produce clear physical reactions as well as psychological ones. Even so, you will find that many orthodox doctors dismiss aromatherapy more quickly than they would homeopathy or herbalism.

Nevertheless, aromatherapy can be useful in both hay fever and asthma. Although you can buy aromatherapy oils in many High Street stores these days, massage is an important part of the treatment. Hence you will be best treated if you visit an aromatherapy practitioner who knows which oils are best suited to your condition and can also perform the necessary massage.

Aromatherapy preparations that use camomile and lavender can reduce inflammation. Those that use eucalyptus can cut down on congestion. There are other preparations that reduce stress – and these may be particularly useful for asthma and hay fever sufferers. You can also buy aromatherapy bath oils that reduce stress.

However, aromatherapy does not provide the level of medical care for asthma or hay fever that is claimed by herbalism or homeopathy. You might like therefore to consider aromatherapy as contributing to your overall care. For people with asthma, though, massage with oils may be particularly helpful in relaxing the chest muscles.

You will find aromatherapists listed in Yellow Pages under Aromatherapy. Look for someone who is a member of the International Association of Aromatherapists or who has the letters ITEC after his or her name.

Reflexology

This is another alternative therapy in vogue at the moment. Reflexologists believe that the sole of the foot contains a complete map of the human body within it. By stimulating the appropriate part of the foot you can also cause the corresponding part of the body to be stimulated. Practitioners say that the energy levels of the diseased tissue can be corrected by such stimulation, thus restoring health.

There is very little empirical evidence to support reflexology. However, it follows the same principles of acupuncture, the technique of which are now widely accepted in orthodox medicine. Nevertheless, most doctors dismiss reflexology as bunkum. Even so, many people report improvements in their condition after visiting a reflexologist.

People are also convinced of the value of reflexology because its practitioners will not even ask what illness you suffer from. They detect your condition simply by manipulating your feet. The fact that reflexologists can diagnose accurately in many instances, just by rubbing and pressing on a patient's foot, is enough to convince them of the effect of this alternative treatment.

You may find that reflexology takes a long time to achieve a significant result. You will need to persevere with the treatments because the therapy appears to work best when taken in small doses over a period of time.

Again, a suitably qualified reflexologist will be of most use. You can find reflexologists in Yellow Pages listed under Reflexology or Therapists.

Summary

Though herbalism and homeopathy are those most widely used, there is a range of other therapies available for the treatment of asthma and hay fever. Aromatherapy and reflexology may also be helpful, particularly for people with asthma. Other alternative treatments are used less frequently – so finding suitably qualified practitioners may be difficult.

If you want to consider alternative therapies, do discuss it first with your doctor. Unlike other medical conditions that benefit from alternative medicine, asthma is potentially fatal. You must not therefore undertake any new treatments without proper discussion.

Most doctors and alternative practitioners will advise that alternative therapies are best considered for preventative treatment rather than to deal with an actual attack.

Remember that an asthma attack can be life-threatening. Whilst an alternative medicine might help get rid of the attack, you would be gambling to some extent if you did not use your bronchodilator to improve your condition immediately. Hence alternative therapies for asthma are preventions, not cures.

Alternative medicines can be used more widely for hay fever as they are unlikely to do you any harm.

Chapter 7
Children and Teenagers with Asthma

Children suffering from asthma or hay fever have special problems.

The symptoms can interfere with their social life, their academic performance and their general outlook. Their treatment can make them feel odd and other children may even taunt them because of their condition.

Children

A higher proportion of children suffer from asthma than any other age group. The latest research suggests that one in every seven youngsters has asthma; and the figures continue to rise. Just ten years ago, the incidence was one in every ten children. According to many experts, pollution – particularly vehicle exhaust fumes – is the reason for this increase.

Many children are first diagnosed as having asthma at around the age of five; and starting school seems to be the time when wheeziness is first noticed. Some are discovered to have asthma at an earlier age, even in infancy.

Babies

Asthma in babies is particularly worrying. Episodes of wheeziness are disturbing to parents as well as to the infants who don't understand what is happening.

Fortunately, the youngest babies do not seem to get asthma attacks as such – only wheeziness. Protection against airway irritation, usually passed on to new-born babies by the mother, wears off in about a year. Therefore, babies can suffer from asthma from the age of one.

Children under four are not usually capable of using an inhaler at all, let alone properly. This means that the management of asthma in young children is often difficult. The medication is often given in the form of a syrup. But getting youngsters to drink their medicine is notoriously difficult.

Also, because the drug isn't being delivered directly to where it is required – the lungs – it takes time to act. Dosages need to be higher than would be used in an inhaler, but not large enough to cause side effects. Since the drug is swallowed, it reaches other tissues in the body and not just the lungs; and this increases the risks of adverse reactions.

To overcome these problems, the doctor may suggest using an inhaler with a spacer device. Alternatively, a nebuliser may be recommended. Even so, both are difficult to use. Children aged about two have a very short attention span – so sitting down with a nebuliser for several minutes is not the easiest task!

For this reason you might like to ask your child's doctor if alternative remedies are possible. Very young children, under the age of two, tend to have only mild asthma. This means that treatments like homeopathy may well be worth trying. Indeed, according to some asthma specialists, such therapy appears to work well in young children.

Pre-school years

Asthma begins to make its presence felt when children grow up a bit and start running around. Four to five is a common age for it to be first diagnosed.

Treating asthma at this age is easier than dealing with infants; but it is not without difficulty. Four year olds can be taught how to use an inhaler properly; but they need to be watched constantly. Inhaler technique can become sloppy when there are so many other interesting activities at playtime.

The asthma may not be fully controlled if the child is allowed to use the inhaler freely and without any discipline.

Equally, if the child is forced to use the inhaler properly, rather than just guided, there is a risk that the child will be made to feel very different to other children. In turn this can lead to deeply rooted psychological problems that will not help the child deal with life – or with asthma in the long term.

The best way to avoid this is for parents of first-time asthma sufferers to treat the use of inhalers as normal. Try not to make the child feel that by using an inhaler he or she is in any way different. Get the child into a routine with the inhaler and keep a check on technique every now and then – but not constantly. In other words, don't allow the child to focus on the inhaler as something too special. It is special of course and can be a life saver; but if a four year old with asthma begins to believe that the inhaler is a life saver, this can have a negative effect on his or her psychological development.

So with toddlers, the key task is to ensure that medication is being delivered to the lungs properly, without making the child feel that there is a terrible problem. At the same time, the child should be made to understand that the condition is serious enough to be respected.

This is a difficult balance for parents to achieve. Some help in walking this tightrope should be available from your GP.

Asthma clinics

Many GPs now hold regular asthma clinics, which are special sessions just for asthma patients.

The clinics are usually run by practice nurses who have been specially trained to deal with asthma problems. A doctor is also often in attendance to deal with special difficulties.

Most of the patients at asthma clinics are children. This means that clinics can provide an additional source of help to parents, who will be able to talk problems over with other parents there.

It is useful to be able to discuss your youngster's condition with others who have encountered and resolved similar difficulties. You will be able to pick up hints and tips on how to get your child to take the medication properly as well as much other practical advice. Added to this, you will be able to discuss matters with the practice nurse and the doctor.

Schoolchildren

The biggest problem with schoolchildren who have asthma lies with the school and not with the children. A survey at the beginning of 1994, published by the National Asthma Campaign, revealed some distressing statistics about schools and the way they handle children who have asthma.

One of the most worrying facts in this nationwide survey was that, in a quarter of all secondary schools, inhalers are taken away from the children and locked in cupboards. This means that 25% of all asthma sufferers over the age of 11 do not have instant access to their own inhalers which could save their lives.

One mother interviewed in the survey said:

When Ellen first started at the school, it was the policy to keep all asthma inhalers in the teachers' desks. But the school then decided this wasn't safe and that all the medication should be kept in the staff room on the first floor.

This meant that if children were having difficulty breathing in class or outdoors, they would have to find someone to go and get their inhaler for them. Or they would have to climb the stairs themselves, gasping for breath all the way.

Despite approaching the school to talk about adopting a more sensible policy towards asthma, the asthma medication remained in the same place and we decided to move Ellen to another school.

Ellen was just eight years old at the time. This case indicates that, even though the survey found that secondary schools are particularly likely to lock up inhalers, primary schools also carry out this senseless practice. There is nothing to be gained by locking up inhalers and there is a great deal to be lost.

Firstly, teachers are putting a child's health and possibly his or her life at risk. Also, by so doing, the teachers are over medicalising the condition and making asthmatic youngsters feel that they are different from everyone else in the class. In other words, it confirms that they are special in an odd sort of way. That's not a very sensible way of helping a child to learn to grow and develop normally.

In addition, such children tend to feel isolated and stressed. They worry that they will become seriously ill if they have an attack. They feel that their health is threatened; and they sometimes believe that they may die. If an attack does occur, their usual sense of panic is heightened dramatically.

Added to all this, locking away the inhalers makes other children in the class believe that those with asthma are different and peculiar. This in turn alters their behaviour towards them.

Children whose inhalers are locked away at school are thus being forced to believe there is something wrong with them – something less tangible than just straightforward asthma.

Teachers seem to believe that the drugs used for treating asthma are dangerous and far more damaging than other items readily available in schools. On the contrary, asthma drugs are very safe indeed. They are so safe that children are allowed to use them for self-medication. Indeed, children are allowed to adjust their dosage according to their own requirements, after explanations from their doctor and practice nurse. Even a teacher would not be allowed to alter the dosage for self-medication of any other safe drug, such as an antibiotic for example.

True, asthma inhalers should not be used by people who do not have asthma. But that's not a reason to lock them away. The child with asthma is hardly likely to pass the inhaler around the class for a quick puff by all and sundry. Equally, those with asthma just don't let the inhaler out of their sight! They know they might need it. Hence it is not likely that an inhaler will fall into unauthorised hands.

Quite frankly, schoolteachers who lock up inhalers are not adequately performing their duty of care to the children.

Thankfully, three quarters of all schools do allow children to keep hold of their inhalers. Nevertheless, with an estimated one million schoolchildren suffering from asthma, some 250,000 of them are not allowed to retain their inhalers during the day. Clearly, if your child has asthma you need to investigate the school's policy and decide carefully what you need to do if it won't allow your youngster to keep the inhaler.

Happily, most of the schools surveyed by the National Asthma Campaign admit that they know very little about asthma and agree that they would like to know much more. Indeed, fewer than ten per cent of teachers admit to any knowledge of asthma drugs. A further eight out of ten teachers say that they want special information on how to deal with pupils who have asthma.

This knowledge gap has been resolved by the National Asthma Campaign which has produced a special Schools Pack of information. If your child's school appears to be in the Dark Ages as far as asthma is concerned, you ought to obtain a pack for it. The National Asthma Campaign can be reached on 071-226 2260.

Teenagers

Teenagers with asthma can experience special problems of their own.

Often they see friends who also have asthma get better, with fewer symptoms and fewer attacks – some may not even need an inhaler any more. But they continue to get symptoms and definitely do need their inhalers. This suggests that they are different. They worry that their health is in danger and that they have a very serious form of asthma.

Asthma varies tremendously from individual to individual. In their case, it is just that they have remained allergic to something and still get the symptoms. There is nothing strange about that. Indeed some people only start to develop allergies when they are teenagers or even adults. A clear explanation to teenagers with asthma may avoid much needless worry.

Unresolved fears may contribute to increased symptoms or to more severe episodes of wheeziness. Hence it is important to give teenagers with asthma the psychological support they need. They should also visit an asthma clinic to be assured that they are in no way special or strange.

There is also another problem encountered by teenagers with asthma. Using an inhaler is thought of as "wet". It is hardly the image that a macho 14-year-old boy would like to project – nor, for that matter, an attractive 16-year-old girl trying to impress her first boyfriend. As a result, teenagers tend to neglect their treatment programmes; and that spells trouble. This is often why teenage youngsters suffer badly from asthma symptoms.

There is no doubt that non-compliance with treatment, responsible for many asthma attacks and episodes of wheeziness, is most frequent during teenage years – it simply doesn't fit the right image. As well as psychological support, teenagers also need a guiding hand to ensure that they take their medication properly.

This can be difficult. A rebellious youngster may not take medication if you, as a parent, insist that it is important. Once again, this is where asthma clinics can help. There, teenagers and older youngsters will tell each other about the need to medicate. Teenagers who are unlikely to do what mum and dad tell them, will be more willing to do what their friends recommend. So use peer pressure, if you can, to get your teenager to take the medicine properly.

Growing out of asthma

One of the biggest worries of parents is that their child will not grow out of asthma. The theory that asthma is a disease of childhood, that cures itself on growing up, is only partly true.

Many youngsters do indeed suffer fewer and fewer attacks as they get older. Their episodes of wheeziness also become less frequent and they feel less chest tightness. With this gradual reduction in symptoms, they are able to reduce their medication as well. Eventually, they no longer need their inhalers.

Such children have not grown out of asthma and their airways remain hyperactive. What appears to have happened is that their ability to cope with the allergy has increased. They have grown away from the symptoms – but their asthma is still there, lurking in the background.

For many youngsters this is the end result. Their bodies have learned to control the condition. They no longer get symptoms and they don't need medication. They appear to have grown out of asthma.

However, it is clear that many children do not grow out of asthma completely. Some people who had asthma as children begin to get symptoms again later in life. This indicates that the allergy was not cured and that the asthma did not go away.

For children who do appear to grow out of asthma, there is always the risk that the condition may reappear later in life. This doesn't mean that they need to change their lifestyles. It simply means that they may suffer symptoms once again in adult life. If they do, they will know how to cope.

Happily, many children do lose their episodes of wheeziness and can do without medication. They never need it again for the rest of their lives. Although their bodies still have asthma, biologically, they are not aware of it.

Explaining asthma

Worrying about children not growing out of asthma is just one concern of parents. Another is how to explain to children that they have a serious and potentially life-threatening disease – yet they shouldn't get too disturbed by it?

There is no easy answer to this; but the asthma clinic can be a tremendous source of support and advice. By visiting an asthma clinic, your child will be able to talk to other youngsters – which will help him or her to understand the condition better.

It is clear that being vague and talking around the subject doesn't help. Children are much more capable of understanding than adults often believe. So, tell your child the truth. Explain the way normal lungs work. Explain that his or her airways don't work quite as efficiently and that some help may be needed to get them working properly again. Even some basic allergy explanations will be understood by youngsters.

Encourage your child to consider himself or herself as a normal individual with a potentially serious condition. In the past, children with asthma were cocooned and separated from other youngsters. They grew up thinking themselves abnormal – which they are not! They are normal children with over-sensitive immune systems and rather sensitive lungs.

Chapter 8
Children and Teenagers with Hay Fever

Incidence

Hay fever is mostly an adult condition. However, children can succumb to the symptoms; and teenagers are the most likely to be affected.

Exams

The biggest problem for teenage sufferers from hay fever is having to cope with exams at a time of year when their symptoms are at their worst. Youngsters may not do so well in their exams if they are suffering from hay fever symptoms at the same time.

Teenagers with hay fever need to understand their condition as soon as possible. This means that they need rapid diagnosis to determine which allergens are responsible for their condition. The sooner they find out, the better. They will then be able to minimise their symptoms and manage their summertime exams more easily.

If possible, the precise allergen that affects them should be pin-pointed. If this is not practicable, every attempt should be made to control the symptoms. This means considering alternative therapies as well as traditional remedies.

Youngsters may still have problems at exam time, even after identification of the allergen and taking appropriate treatment – for the stress of exams can reduce the performance of their immune systems. This means that treatment adequate to control symptoms in normal circumstances will not be powerful enough when it comes to exam time. Hence, teenagers with hay fever really need to take preventive action before the exam season begins.

This starts with telling the teacher – honesty is the best policy. Explain that hay fever is a problem and that special care may be required around exam time. Such care could include taking the exam in a special room, where the windows and doors are closed to prevent any pollens from coming in. This may mean that a teenager with hay fever will need to take the exam alone with a separate invigilator. Ask also if the exam room can have an air filter in it. These are portable machines that can extract pollens from the surrounding atmosphere. They can also be useful at home when placed in the bedroom or study of teenagers suffering from hay fever.

The necessary arrangements can be made if the school is told well in advance – particularly those involving the Examining Board.

It's also a good idea to consult your GP if serious hay fever is likely to affect examination performance. Your doctor can provide a medical certificate which the Examination Board can take into account when marking the papers.

Another good ploy is to see if the exam can be taken at another time of year other than in early summer when hay fever is most troubling. Many exams are possible in January, when pollens are very low. You may need to arrange this well in advance so that extra tuition is available. Taking an exam six months earlier than you might expect can involve a lot of additional pressure. Only by talking to the teachers can you work out whether this is a viable option.

Chapter 9
Stress and the Breathing System

Stress is a significant problem for people with breathing difficulties. Whether you have asthma or hay fever, stress will make your condition worse. Stress, though, is important; we all need some stress. When people talk about stress what they really mean is excess stress.

The idea of stress as a medical problem was first introduced in the 1920s by a medical student from Prague. However it was not until the mid-1970s, when that same student had become a professor in Montreal, that his concept of stress became integrated into modern medical thinking.

Essentially, stress is the response by the body to various outside demands made on it. Something that frightens us, for example, is a stressor; and the biological reaction which our body produces in response to it is the stress.

Stress differs between individuals. What frightens or worries you and produces stress symptoms, may not frighten your next door neighbour who will therefore not suffer any symptoms.

The biology of stress

Your body reacts in essentially the same way whenever any stressor appears. Your brain is first involved; this decides very rapidly whether or not the difficulty you are confronting is a stressor. Once it has calculated that a stressor is present, chemicals are released within the body to prepare you to deal with the threat. Like the body's immune system, the reaction to stress is another defence mechanism to ensure survival.

The main chemical released is adrenaline which comes from a gland situated above each kidney. Adrenaline is a hormone – a chemical messenger that instructs other parts of the body to do certain things. Adrenaline orchestrates a major change within your body to enable you to deal with the stressor. Essentially, it prepares you for a fight or flight response. Your body is prepared either to confront the stressor head on, or else to get away from it as fast as it can.

To achieve this, hormonal changes ensure that blood is diverted away from your intestines to the muscles of your legs and chest – more oxygen is delivered to the muscles needed to deal with the stressor. But because the blood is moved away from your intestines, digestion has to be halted or slowed down considerably.

The stress reaction makes you breathe more rapidly to improve oxygen supply. This helps get rid of the build-up of carbon dioxide and ensures that increased amounts of oxygen become available to the blood.

Chemicals which help blood to clot are increased – so that your body can effect a quick repair if the stressor causes a real physical problem.

There is an urgent need to empty the bladder immediately, even if it isn't full, so that you are better prepared to deal with the stressor. The kidneys also stop processing urine so that you won't be disturbed by the need to pop to the loo in the middle of the fight or flight.

Another hormonal effect is to provide a readily available energy supply by increasing the amount of glucose and fat in your blood. Your blood pressure rises so that this energy can be quickly pumped around the body.

Adrenaline also ensures that the area of your brain that has sexual thoughts is effectively switched off. No risks can be taken and you must be able to face the stressor without wandering off into some erotic fantasy!

The result

The result of all this activity – which takes about two seconds to complete – is a well-honed machine ready either to fight the stressor or to make a rapid escape.

Now, all this is fine if the threat is real. If you are ever faced with a manic hippopotamus roaring down the High Street, your body will be well prepared to run like crazy. You will cope with relative ease because extra energy has been made readily available, your muscles, heart and lungs have been prepared for the effort and your brain has been concentrated to deal with the problem in hand.

But what if the threat is not a manic hippopotamus? What if the stressor is an angry boss at work? Or the worry that you might have asthma on holiday?

Even with those kinds of stressors, adrenaline is released and your body is prepared to cope in exactly the same way.

But because – unlike the disappearance of the hippo – there is no real end to this type of stressor, your body doesn't know when to switch off its fight or flight response. It continues with a higher blood pressure than it needs, your breathing rate is more rapid than necessary, your digestion is slowed down, your kidneys are not working as efficiently as they should, there is too much fat in your bloodstream and your brain's sexual thoughts are much reduced.

Non-real stressors, like worries about asthma, leave your body's chemistry and systems in this altered state.

Stress symptoms

Stress symptoms quickly develop even when stressors are more imaginary than real.

It's probably no surprise that one of the key symptoms of excess stress is a reduction in sexual activity. Your brain switches off its sexual thought processes in order to cope with the stressor.

Indigestion and irritable bowel symptoms are also very common in people with stress. That's because the blood supply to the digestive tract has been reduced, preventing the system from functioning efficiently.

Similarly, the preparation of your muscles for fight or flight leads to feelings of tension that can cause aches and pains.

The most common stress symptoms are:

Irritability
Low sex drive
Tiredness
Indigestion
Nausea
Constipation
Diarrhoea
Dizziness
Headaches
Neck pain
Insomnia
Breathlessness
Chest pain
Sweating
Lack of concentration

As you can see, some of the symptoms of excess stress from non-real stressors are the same as those you get in asthma or hay fever. These include breathlessness, chest pains and headaches.

Stress and asthma

There are two aspects to stress and asthma. Firstly, any additional stress in your life can increase the severity of your asthma symptoms. If you are having a bad day and your asthma is not well-controlled, stress can add to the symptoms by making you more breathless or giving you chest pains as well. Secondly, being stressed and anxious can itself bring on an attack of asthma.

Some people find that they only have asthma attacks when they are under pressure. Those individuals are not allergic to anything; they have asthma attacks simply as a result of stress.

It's important, therefore, for people with asthma to learn to control stress. This will reduce the severity of their symptoms and will also help to lessen the number of stress-induced attacks.

Stress and hay fever

As with asthma, your hay fever will almost certainly get worse if you are stressed.

It has been established that stress makes your body even more susceptible to allergens. So if you are particularly stressed at any time, you may find that your hay fever comes on even though the pollen count is relatively low. Your body is just that much more susceptible to the allergens.

Reducing stress will help you cope with higher pollen counts and will also ensure that your symptoms will be less severe when they do occur.

Stress reduction

Clearly, reducing stress is an important factor in minimising the effects of both hay fever and asthma. If you keep your stress levels low, you will be less likely to have attacks and if you do suffer from them, the symptoms will be less severe.

The main problems which cause stress these days are conflicts. You probably won't be faced with a hippo in the High Street; but you may be faced by one half of your family wanting one thing and the other half wanting something completely different. Or you may find that you need three days to do a particular job that your boss insists must be done in two. Or the teacher at school says the homework must be done tonight, when you have an important session at the youth club.

Most stress is caused by conflict and the biggest single conflict you are likely to face is some kind of pressure on your time.

Time management

The single biggest contribution you can make to reducing stress levels is to manage your time effectively. Time management is essential to your overall well-being. It will reduce your stress symptoms and the severity and frequency of bouts of hay fever or attacks of asthma. Indeed, proper time management can reduce the chances of an asthma attack; being forced to rush from one event to another because of poor time management could in itself bring on wheeziness due to a combination of the exercise and the stress.

When people talk about time management they think of a fancy leather binder with a complicated diary system, accompanied by the endless writing down of absolutely every detail of your day. While such systems are effective, they are not necessary. You don't need a ring binder or a diary system – but just a few sheets of paper on which to write things down so that you can get a clear picture of all the demands on your time.

The first thing to do is to write down all the things you have to do. Put everything on the list, absolutely everything, and don't leave anything out.

Include all work-related items, family tasks and domestic jobs. Write down all your appointments and social engagements. Just jot down everything that you know must be done. You don't have to worry about when the item needs doing. If it's mid-summer and you have just thought of Christmas shopping, shove that on the list as well.

Take your time over this first step. Prepare the list and put it to one side. Go back to it later and add some more items. Repeat this again and again until you are sure everything is there.

Now that you have a list of all the demands on your time, you can begin to make decisions.

Look at your list and mark each item with an A, B or C. Those marked A are the high priority tasks, all absolutely essential. B items are those which need doing, but not so urgently. The items marked C are nice to do if you have the time – but they are not vital.

Now take your A items and list them in order of priority. The one at the top of your list will be the most urgent job to be done. The bottom of your A list will also be important but can wait for a while. Do the same with your B list and your C list. The last item on your C list wouldn't really matter if it was never done at all.

Go back to your A list and give each item a deadline. What is the date by which each job must be done? Buying a birthday present, for example, needs to be completed by the day before the birthday. If you are not sure when an item needs completing, give it a deadline anyway. This discipline will help ensure that everything gets done.

Now go through every item and give it a starting date. It's all very well giving tasks a time for completion, but your stress will rise if you only discover that an item needs doing just before the deadline is about to expire! Work out the starting dates carefully. If, for instance, you normally only take three days to do the Christmas shopping, your start date would be 21st December – that way you will be sure of meeting your deadline.

Having given everything a start date and a completion date, you can now enter things into your diary. Put all the items that need to be done under their start dates. So, for instance, your diary would show "Start Christmas shopping" under 21st December. As you write in each item make sure you put its code letter A, B or C next to it. Also jot down the expected time it will take.

Now your diary will have some pages with items on them and others without. Go to the first page with items on it and look for those coded A. These are going to be the tasks that must be dealt with on that day. If there are a number of them, you can ignore the C items completely and you can relegate the Bs to another day.

Now put specific times against the A items. Say your diary shows the following:

A   Write report on new project (2 hrs)
A   Start analysing sales figures (12 hrs)
A   Go to Steven's school play at 7 pm (3 hrs)
B   Order new computer (10 mins)
B   Discuss new project with planning department (30 mins)
C   Fix the dripping tap in the bathroom. (15 mins)

Let's look at this list. Clearly there are not enough hours in the day to get it all done. The A items are essential, so these must be dealt with – but even they add up to 17 hours! What you need to do is to split the long project up into its stages and then give each of these a start and end time. Hence the "Start analysing sales figures" could become:

Enter new sales figures onto computer (2 hrs)
Print out and read sales figures report (1 hr)
Select best sales area from the printout (1 hr)
Enter the detailed sales figures for this area onto the computer (2 hrs)
Print out and read selected sales figures report (1 hr)
Select best sales executive from the report printout (1 hr)
Print out and read best sales executive's daily figures (1 hr)
Calculate sales commissions (1 hr)
Write and print report on this month's sales (2 hrs).

These are all category A items and can now be entered in the diary; and there will be no problem providing that the last one on the list is done by our deadline. So today's diary might read:

9.00 am .... Write report on new project
11.00 .... Discuss new project with planning department
11.30 .... Coffee break
11.50 .... Order new computer
12.00 noon... Start entering new sales figures onto computer
1.00 pm .... Lunch
2.00 .... Carry on entering new sales figures
3.00 .... Print out and read sales figures
4.00 .... Select best sales area
5.00 .... Go home – need to be home to get ready for school play!
7.00 .... School play.

By writing things down like this, you can be sure that you meet your deadlines. If you didn't work out priorities and break the projects down into small segments, you would start on the big project to get it cleared out of the way and would then not do the other A items. You would probably work right through until the last possible minute and then rush off to the school play, without time for a meal. You'd feel hurried and upset because you hadn't had time to finish the report. You'd also probably end up arguing at home because you only made it to the play at the last minute!

With the more structured approach, you get all the jobs done, meet your deadlines, have more free time to yourself and do not end up with a conflict between work and home.

Time management is about organising your work and home life to provide you with a flexible timetable to avoid conflicts. You do not have to know exactly what is going on in every hour – though our example did to show how to split up a big project.

What is essential is to prioritise all your tasks and then commit them to paper with a start and an end time. Then you no longer have to worry about them and the jobs will get done when they need to be done. Without this approach, you may forget important tasks and will probably do things that are not as important – then you will run out of time.

That will lead to conflict and the end result will be stress and pressure. This will just compound your problem because you will feel ill. Your asthma or hay fever will play up, making you less effective and unable to perform at your peak. That will increase the amount of time you need to do things. Your hay fever will worsen, or you'll have an asthma attack. You'll then need even more time and will feel more stressed. After months like this, you'll say that you feel as if you are on a treadmill!

All of this can be avoided with simple time management – one of the most important ways of reducing excess stress.

Relaxation

Very few people take enough time to relax. They often confuse relaxing with lounging about and watching the TV, or having a gin and tonic after a hard day at work. Neither of these is proper relaxation. Yet there is ample evidence that relaxation reduces stress and improves overall well-being. If you have asthma or hay fever, relaxation will help to reduce the severity of your symptoms.

Proper relaxation will allow your mind and body to relax together. Once you have learned the techniques, you will be able to use them when under pressure. For example, if your boss at work suddenly springs a surprise on you, a few simple relaxation exercises will help you to control your stress and prevent your body from reacting to the stressor.

It is a good idea to devote half an hour each day for learning to relax. At first you will probably find the relaxation techniques unusual; but with practice you will do them automatically and derive much benefit from them.

When your half-hour relaxation period arrives, take yourself off to a quiet room. Your bedroom is probably a good place. Make sure you will not be disturbed. Take the phone off the hook, switch off the TV, and tell the children to keep downstairs!

Now ensure that you are in comfortable clothes. You won't want any tight belts or jumpers that constrict, for instance. Many people find that they prefer to be naked when relaxing – but if so, ensure the room is warm or you will not be able to relax properly.

You will probably find it easier to relax if there are no bright lights. Many people find that they need to have the room in darkness when first trying relaxation techniques.

Lay down on the bed and get comfortable. Close your eyes and concentrate your mind on your feet; imagine they are getting heavy. You will then begin to notice that your feet are feeling warm and heavy. You may find that alternately contracting and relaxing the muscles a few times will help. Once your feet have become heavy, move your attention to your legs. Repeat this exercise for all other parts of the body, ending with your face. Take your time; the whole process should last about 20 minutes.

Yoga is another well-established method of relaxation. Yoga has been studied medically; and it has been demonstrated that high blood pressure can be lowered by performing yoga exercises. Breathing control is a very important aspect of yoga technique.

To learn yoga properly you should attend classes. Many education authorities provide evening classes in yoga at local schools. There are also clubs run by the Yoga for Health Foundation. Your local library will be able to tell you if there is such a club in your area.

Breathing control techniques

Breathing control is particularly useful for people with asthma. Not only will it help to reduce stress overall, it can also be of practical help when you feel wheezy.

Breathing techniques are also useful for people with hay fever. They help to cut down stress; and stress affects the immune system and makes you more vulnerable to pollen.

Breathing techniques work well when you need to relax quickly. For example, suppose that the boss has just come in and demanded that you do some work immediately; and you feel stressed because you cannot do what is required. You probably can't rush off to a darkened room, strip off your clothes and have a 20 minute relaxation session! What you can do in the office though is to perform some simple breathing control techniques that will help keep you calm and diminish the effects of the stress.

The principle behind all breathing control techniques is "control".

When you need instant relaxation, breathe slowly. You may find this easier to do by breathing through your mouth. You need to perform a half swallow! Restrict the space at the back of your throat by starting to swallow. Then breathe in slowly through your mouth. The air will rush into your lungs rapidly because you have narrowed your throat. Take a deep breath as slowly as you can; then let the air out slowly. Repeat this a number of times and you will feel more relaxed. If you can, use this relaxing breathing technique every morning and night.

However, do not do this exercise if you have to strain to breathe, if you already feel wheezy or if it takes any effort.

Another useful technique is abdominal breathing. This is where your breathing is definitely under the control of your diaphragm. Your diaphragm is a sheet of muscular tissue that separates your chest from your abdomen. It moves up and down as you breathe.

To try abdominal breathing lie down on your bed and relax. Your head should be slightly raised on a pillow. Place your hands just at the top of your abdomen, below your rib cage. Now try to breathe by pushing your abdomen out with your diaphragm. Take a slow, deep breath, then slowly let it out again by pushing your diaphragm upwards. After a while you will get used to using your diaphragm for breathing; many people with asthma find that using this breathing technique also helps when they are wheezy or having an attack.

Exercise

Statistics show that fewer and fewer people exercise on a regular basis. However, regular exercise does more than keep you fit; it helps reduce stress.

The reason is that exercise stimulates the release of chemicals in the brain called endorphins. These chemicals lead to a generally relaxed feeling – and you get an emotional high when you produce a great amount of them. Indeed, exercise can become addictive for some people as it produces the kind of euphoric feeling that you get with some drugs; they lead to the release of endorphins as well.

Regular exercise will undoubtedly reduce stress and also be beneficial to your overall health. Unfortunately, exercise with asthma can be a problem. Many people suffer from exercise-induced asthma (see Chapter 12) and others become wheezy after a bout of exercise. But you can benefit from the stress-reducing effects of exercise if you are careful. Take your preventive treatment just before you exercise. And wear comfortable, loose fitting clothes that will not restrict your chest. If you suffer from hay fever don't exercise when the pollen count is high.

Swimming is the best form of exercise for someone with asthma or hay fever. The warm moist air improves breathing and the buoyancy of the water helps your chest. You must swim, rather than splash about in the water, for your body needs to exercise. You need to increase your heart rate and feel as though you have made some effort!

Do not rush into exercise if you are otherwise lazy. Take things slowly and build up your performance. If you are starting an exercise programme from scratch, see your GP first. You won't be talked out of it by your doctor, or given a list of reasons why you shouldn't do it. But you will be told how much exercise you can do, given your own particular circumstances.

Walking is the next best thing to swimming. Three 20 minute walks each week is all you need. Many people also find that at the end of a tiring day, a 20 minute walk around the block makes them feel more relaxed and ready for a good night's sleep.

Other stress reduction techniques

You may still be stressed even if you do manage your time well, relax, take up exercise and learn breathing techniques.

Your diet may be contributing; and it has been shown that a well-balanced diet can help to reduce stress.

You should also consider whether any problems in your life need resolving.

Is your stress due to worries about your marriage? Are you under stress because you fear redundancy? You should not let concerns like these get bottled up inside you. Doing so increases your stress. Talk about any worries you may have – this helps resolve them. You may also learn that they are not as serious as you thought.

There are a number of ways you can talk things out. You can start with your family and have regular talk sessions. Or you can use a friend's shoulder to cry on. If you would feel embarrassed by this, try a local support group. Many areas now have groups of people who simply get together to talk over their fears and concerns; your local library will have a list of suitable groups. If you cannot find anyone with whom to talk things over, you might benefit from seeing a counsellor or therapist. Choose a properly qualified individual listed under Counselling and Advice in Yellow Pages.

Another technique that helps reduce stress is to follow a creative hobby like gardening, art, needlework and so on. This will take your mind off other issues and give you something else to think about. Don't choose a hobby that involves contests or competitions, for that will just increase your stress levels. So if you like gardening as a way of relieving stress, don't enter your marrows in the summer fete contest!

A simple smile is another way of relieving stress. Try to smile as often as you can. It makes you feel happier and it prompts other people to respond to you more positively – in turn helping you feel better.

Also, try kissing more frequently! Studies have shown that people who kiss each other regularly have lower levels of stress than others who do not. The kissing actually stimulates the release of endorphins – which are the stress-reducing chemicals also produced in exercise.

Chapter 10
Living with Asthma and Hay Fever

Even if your asthma or hay fever is being treated properly and you are taking some kind of alternative medicine and you have ensured that your stress levels are at their lowest, there are still other practical things you can do to help relieve your condition.

Most of these are simple day-to-day things – precautions that you can take quite easily. They will help you keep your symptoms to a minimum and will make life more bearable.

Avoiding allergens

The simplest and surest way to keep out of trouble is to stay as far away from the allergen as possible – that is if you know which one causes your symptoms.

Don't, for example, go for walks in the woods during pollination if you know that your hay fever is caused by a particular kind of tree pollen. Consider parting with the cat if its fur causes your asthma. Get someone else to cut the grass if mowing the lawn brings on attacks of hay fever.

In other words, if you know the actual cause of your hay fever or asthma, avoiding it will have a significant impact on your day-to-day life and you will be far less likely to suffer from attacks of symptoms.

However, what is often the biggest problem can't be avoided very easily – or so it seems. That is the house dust mite.

House dust mites

The droppings of house dust mites are one of the commonest triggers for asthma attacks. They also cause a form of hay fever known as perennial rhinitis – with it you feel as though you have a permanent cold.

House dust mites are present in every home. You don't have to be especially dirty to have them. Even the Queen has house dust mites!

House dust mites are microscopic creatures, which live by eating human skin. They are likely to exist wherever there are people.

We each shed tiny fragments of skin every day in the form of millions of skin cells. They become loosened by movement, by touching objects, by stroking our skin, by the rubbing of clothes against our skin and so on. In fact a significant proportion of the dust in your house consists of skin fragments.

Though human skin particles are usually dry when shed, they will absorb moisture under the right conditions – especially in a damp or humid house. This is when the trouble starts, for the house dust mite just loves moist, dead, human skin. It thrives on such food. If it's warm as well, the house dust mite is in its element!

Your bed is probably the warmest and most humid place in your house. That's also where you shed most of your skin for you thrash about at night – everyone changes their sleeping position on average more than 30 times during the night! All of that movement rubs skin off your body and it collects in the bedding. Added to that, you are nice and warm in bed and your body is lightly sweating. That all provides lovely moist conditions for the house dust mites to have a field day!

The dust mites defaecate as they feed off your skin in your bed. They produce pellets of dung which are extremely dry and very tiny – only about one fiftieth of a millimetre wide. Their dryness enables them to survive for many years and their microscopic size allows them to float about in the air, where you can easily breathe them in.

Consider that the average house dust mite can produce 20 pellets a day and that they live for up to six months. Also that each little mite can produce 840 pellets of dung, and the female can lay 300 eggs, during its lifetime. With about two million of these little mites in a double bed, you can see that the potential for breathing in the allergen – the droppings – is substantial.

But there are some practical steps you can take to reduce the problem.

The bedroom

The main production area for house dust mite droppings is your own bed. You should try and limit the potential for the dust mite there as much as you can.

The first step you can take is to reduce the temperature of your bedroom. It's nice to have a lovely warm room when you wake up in the morning, but you could find yourself wheezing and sneezing as a result of a night of frantic mite activity. Ideally, keep the temperature as cool as you can accept; about 16 degrees Celsius is usually tolerable.

Another factor in the bedroom is humidity. Central heating provides a nice warm house and reduces humidity. That may seem good at first sight. But to compensate for the reduced humidity, and to ensure improved efficiency of the central heating system, you probably keep the windows closed. This lack of ventilation results in an increase of humidity.

One way of reducing the humidity of your bedroom is to sleep with the window open. Granny was right when she said you should always sleep with an open window. This helps to reduce the humidity of the room and also lowers the temperature; both of these will limit the number of house dust mites.

Granny also said that it is important to air your bed daily. That's true too. If you make your bed each morning, you will simply cocoon the house dust mite back into its nice warm atmosphere. It will then continue to chomp away on your left-over bits of skin and will produce plenty of fresh droppings for you to breathe in when you get back into bed the following night.

Throw back the sheets each morning, brush off the bed, shake the pillow and leave the bed unmade. It may not impress your neighbours if you show them around, but it will be a nasty shock for the mites. Get someone else to deal with the bedding if you suffer from asthma or perennial rhinitis; for shaking the bedding yourself will cause you to breathe in air that is laden with dust mite droppings – and that could lead to an attack of symptoms.

The bed itself also needs attention. Bedding should be changed as frequently as possible – for keeping sheets and pillowcases on your bed for long periods simply invites the mites to thrive. Also, make sure that you wash the pillows, the blankets and the duvet regularly. Recent studies show that a pillow that hasn't been washed could have up to 10% of its weight made up of house dust mites and human skin! By washing pillows and bedding you will be getting rid of the mites and their eggs as well as disposing of those allergy-causing droppings.

However, the mites will still be living in the bed itself. So every time you change the sheets, you should clean and turn the mattress.

You might also want to consider special protective covers for the mattress. You can now buy such covers from High Street chemists and by mail order. In a recent leaflet on air pollution in the home, the British Lung Foundation (a national charity dedicated to improving life for people with any lung condition) recommended these special coverings because mites cannot pass through them.

In essence, such mattress covers and pillowcases provide a barrier between you and the house dust mite. As you shed skin during the night, the house dust mites in your mattress cannot get through to nibble away at it.

However, the mites will still be living in the pillows and the other bedding. To solve this, you can buy anti-allergy pillows and duvets that incorporate special materials to inhibit the house dust mite. Such bedding is not cheap though. An anti-allergy pillow costs around £25, compared to about £5 for an ordinary pillow. Also, a single mattress cover can be as much as £45. If you were to buy two anti-allergy pillows, a mattress cover and a special duvet for a double bed you would be spending around £250.

Even if you do spend this amount, there will still be house dust mites in your bedroom. They will be breeding in the carpet. As you walk around you shed skin particles into the carpet and create a cloud of dust every time you place your foot on the floor. This propels the house dust mite faeces into the air where you breathe them in. So, limiting the house dust mites in your bed will help; but your bedroom will still contain some mites.

One way to further reduce the mite population in your bedroom is to remove the carpet and have a polished, boarded or linoleum floor. This is not the environment that the house dust mite likes – it is cooler and less moist. When you walk around there will be much smaller clouds of dust than with a carpet – so less allergen is propelled into the air. You will also be able to sponge the floor regularly and wipe away many of the mites and their dung.

But even if you accomplish all these things in the bedroom, the rest of your house will still contain dust mites.

The rest of the house

You can help to reduce the dust mite population throughout your house in a number of ways.

You can resort to polished wooden floors – but this might not be to your taste. So perhaps you could consider keeping windows open more frequently to reduce the humidity. If that's not practical, you could buy a dehumidifier to extract particles of moisture from the air and so reduce the likelihood of house dust mite activity.

One of the best ways of getting rid of house dust mites is to clean thoroughly and regularly. You should make sure that you clean the house with the windows open. That way, much of the dust you throw into the air when you clean can escape outside. Also clean the carpets first and then do the polishing. The dust and the mites you throw into the air from the carpet will settle on the surfaces of objects you want to polish. This means you will get rid of more dust mites if you polish after cleaning the carpets.

Cleaning carpets is one of the biggest problems for sufferers of asthma and hay fever. The pellets of dust mite dung are pushed into the air when you brush carpets, so use a carpet sweeper or a vacuum cleaner.

Also, don't be fooled into thinking that a vacuum cleaner will get rid of your dust mites – it won't! A typical vacuum cleaner can only filter out particles about twice as large as their pellets of dung. The result is that the dust mite droppings are sucked into the vacuum cleaner and then thrown straight back into the air, ready for you to breathe in. Indeed, The Lancet published an article in 1990 which said that conventional vacuum cleaning cannot be recommended for dust mite control in the homes of asthmatics.

You may have seen advertisements for special vacuum cleaners, especially for people with asthma and hay fever. These have been tested in clinical trials and shown to be remarkably effective in reducing dust mites and their droppings. These vacuum cleaners contain very special filters that can trap particles as small as the dust mite dung pellets.

Researchers at Southampton University are now developing special fibres, based on the way these filters work, that could spell disaster for dust mites. This is still experimental; but it suggests that further help is on the way for allergy sufferers.

In the meantime, a special vacuum cleaner may be the answer – if you are prepared to pay the price of around £450.

Do you need to take all these steps to reduce house dust mites?

Whether you need to buy an expensive vacuum cleaner, rid your bedroom of carpets and use special bedding depends only on whether or not you are allergic to house dust mite droppings.

Although an estimated eight out of ten people with asthma are allergic to house dust mites and many others suffer permanently from hay fever symptoms as a result of these pests, not everyone with symptoms is allergic to them. One in every five people with asthma is not allergic to house dust mites and has another cause of their asthma.

So, taking all these actions – and particularly spending a great deal of money on special cleaners and bedding – may be unnecessary. Only consider doing it if you are definitely allergic to house dust mite droppings.

Before you launch into a major assault on your bedroom and spend some of your savings on special equipment, get your doctor to confirm that your allergy is due to the house dust mite. Your doctor can check the source of your allergy by using a simple skin test. The chances are that you will be allergic to the house dust mite faeces, particularly if you have asthma. But check first before you spend any money.

Your diet

You are what you eat, so the saying goes; and people with asthma and hay fever should pay attention to their diet.

One particular problem for people with asthma is an inadequate amount of Vitamin B12. This vitamin is essential for the production of new cells, particularly red blood cells. It is found only in animal sources of food, especially liver, kidneys, and dairy produce. Also, we produce some of it ourselves in our intestines as a result of bacteria that reside there. Even so, this is not enough for our normal functioning. We need Vitamin B12 in our diets to maintain our bodies in peak condition. Unlike some vitamins, Vitamin B12 cannot be stored, so we need to take some in every day.

Research has shown that you need to have the right level of acid in your stomach in order to absorb Vitamin B12. We all naturally produce hydrochloric acid in our stomachs, which is an essential part of our digestive process. But people with asthma often have lower levels of hydrochloric acid. This means that they are less efficient at absorbing Vitamin B12.

Injections of Vitamin B12 in very high doses have been shown to help people with asthma. If you have asthma, it is probably wise to ensure that you get a good supply of Vitamin B12 by eating plenty of foodstuffs that contain it.

Dairy produce may be a problem for some people with asthma for they may be allergic to cows' milk and its products like cheese. In this instance, you might need to consider vitamin supplements. You may also need to include folic acid in these supplements as this helps to increase the absorption of Vitamin B12.

Other vitamins are also important. If you have hay fever, or have had episodes of wheeziness, you will need a healthy body to get your system back to normal. The irritation in the lungs or the lining of the nose will mean that the tissues need repairing and this can only be done effectively if your body has a rich supply of vitamins and minerals. For this reason, people with asthma and hay fever should ensure that they have a well-balanced diet that is rich in vitamins and minerals.

You can achieve a high level of the required nutrients by eating varied foodstuffs regularly. You should eat three meals a day. Starting with a high fibre breakfast cereal is particularly important for it helps fill you up and stops you from snacking during the morning. But more than that, high fibre cereals are packed with essential vitamins. Be sure to eat at lunch time for this boosts your flagging energy levels and also contributes to your vitamin intake.

Try to have fresh foods whenever possible for these are packed with vitamins. The longer you store food, the fewer the vitamins. So eat foods as fresh as possible. Also, do not boil the vitamins out of food when you cook it. Light cooking is best.

Eat the foods straight after they have been cooked; leaving food to stand also depletes their vitamin content. One other tip, eat at least four slices of wholemeal or granary bread each day. The fibre will help your digestive system and the bread is also rich in vitamins.

Consider a vitamin supplement if you can't achieve all the above. Your doctor will tell you they are not necessary. True, they are not necessary to avoid vitamin deficiency diseases; we simply don't get scurvy or beri beri anymore! But what medical science is only just beginning to realise, is that these vitamin deficiency diseases are just the endpoint of significant depletion of vitamins in the diet.

Reduced levels of vitamins can cause a wide range of effects. Hence many people who lead a busy life and who cannot eat fresh foods regularly three times a day, may well need general vitamin supplements. For people with an allergy, such supplementation may be particularly important in helping the body to recover from attacks of symptoms.

Indeed, studies have suggested that very large doses of Vitamin C supplements can have a significant impact on hay fever symptoms.

There is only one warning about vitamin supplements. You should never take more than the recommended dose for Vitamins A and D. Too much of these vitamins can result in overdose symptoms. This is particularly important for pregnant women. So, if you do think you need vitamin supplements, read the label on the bottle carefully and only take the recommended amounts. Combined with an average diet you will be getting sufficient of the essential vitamins and minerals.

Peak flow measurements

You can change your diet and get rid of house dust mites, but you will never completely get rid of your susceptibility to asthma. Your lungs will always be vulnerable to a reduction in their airways and you could suffer from episodes of wheeziness.

For this reason, doctors now recommend regular measurement of the Peak Expiratory Flow (PEF) as an excellent way of monitoring the effectiveness of your control measures and predicting the likelihood of an attack. Peak Expiratory Flow is explained in Chapter 2. That way you can prevent many asthma attacks by taking appropriate avoiding action.

Peak flow meters are simple to use. They are tube-shaped devices with a scale on one side on which is shown the amount of air that passes from your lungs through the instrument.

Your practice nurse will instruct you how to use the meter properly. In essence you take a full breath in, hold it for a second or two, place the mouthpiece of the Peak Flow Meter in your mouth and close your lips around it. Then blow out as fully and as fast as you can. You then read the measurement on the scale on the side of the tube.

It's a good idea to do this three times to make sure that you get an accurate reading. Another useful tip is to take a reading in the morning and another one at night. Asthma is a condition that is affected by the time of day, so twice-daily readings will help establish a clearer picture of your particular condition.

You should keep a written record of your PEF readings. This will help you spot when your breathing worsens and will give your doctor a clearer picture of what is happening.

The readings you record will help you understand your condition better and will enable you to tailor your treatment more precisely. In many instances, they will detect a worsening of your condition far sooner than will your own feelings and symptoms. You can then adjust your treatment in advance to avoid attacks.

If you haven't got a Peak Flow Meter, ask your doctor; they are available on the NHS.

Watching the weather

Watching the TV weather reports, or listening to them on the radio, can be very helpful to sufferers from hay fever or asthma.

The weather broadcasters give warnings about levels of pollen and pollution. Those with hay fever may want to avoid going out when pollen counts are high. Similarly, the amount of pollution in the air can affect asthma sufferers very badly.

Air quality is now measured in the UK, though there is much controversy about how this is done, and these measurements are given in broad terms by the weather broadcasters. Poor air quality means there are plenty of pollutants in the air which could worsen your asthma.

Another useful piece of information provided by the weather experts is the temperature, particularly wind chill factors. Asthma can easily be triggered by blasts of cold air. So keeping an eye on the weather could prevent your going out in nasty, cold, windy conditions. That way you will reduce the chances of an attack.

Coping with attacks

An asthma attack is a frightening experience. It can often lead to panic in someone with asthma; and it is deeply disturbing to watch.

Make sure that your family and friends know what to do if you have an attack of asthma. You can also take some steps to make sure that your symptoms subside quickly.

The first thing to do is always to take your treatment as prescribed. Your doctor will explain how much medicine to take when symptoms are very severe. This will be tailored to your own individual circumstances.

During an attack you will probably find it most comfortable to sit at a table, leaning forward slightly and resting on your elbows. Anything that distracts you from the attack, such as TV, will help.

It's easy to say, but more difficult to do – try not to panic and keep as calm as possible. The stress caused by being in a state of panic can worsen the attack.

Your family should know that, even though they may be distraught, they shouldn't panic either. They should be sure to call your doctor and prepare your nebuliser – if that is needed. They could also open a window if the room is warm and the outside air is not too cold. Your family should also loosen any tight clothing you are wearing. They should keep a close eye on you but not fuss too much so as not to increase your already high stress levels!

Chapter 11
Exercise

Exercise is good for everyone. It promotes good health, reduces the chance of heart disease and keeps your body fit and supple. Exercise helps you to avoid many of the complications of old age – but it can be troublesome for people with asthma or hay fever.

As was explained in Chapter 10, exercise can play an important part in helping to reduce stress and so keep the immune system in shape, reducing the likelihood of symptoms. Gone are the days when children would arrive at school with a note from their parents saying they can't take part in games because they suffer from asthma.

Indeed, with well-controlled asthma, many sports teachers wouldn't even know that some of their pupils suffer from the condition. Unfit youngsters often puff and blow more than the kids with asthma – not because their lungs are unwell, but simply because they themselves are unfit. Even so, asthma, hay fever and exercise often do not mix.

Exercise-induced asthma

Many asthma attacks come on immediately after exercise. Some people only discover they have asthma as a result of an attack occurring after playing some sport.

Exercise-induced asthma may be particularly worrying since the attacks can be severe. Most people get "puffed" after strenuous exercise; but those with asthma can become quite seriously ill.

Exercise-induced asthma is recognised as a special problem by the medical profession – but it is no different from other forms of asthma. It is special only because it can bring on such severe attacks. It also indicates that the individual's condition is not being properly controlled by medicines, making necessary a re-evaluation of the treatment programme. Even so, exercise-induced asthma is merely an asthma attack triggered by the exercise.

What appears to happen in exercise-induced asthma is the irritation of the airways by cold air rushing into the lungs as you breathe more quickly.

It is natural to breathe deeply and quickly during exercise; and it seems that the rush of cold air can trigger an attack in susceptible individuals.

The airways need to be in a hyperactive state, usually as a result of contact with an allergen. But this contact is not sufficient in itself to cause an attack. The inrush of cold air then tips the balance and the attack follows.

Because cold air is the culprit, winter sports are not a good idea for some people with asthma. But if your condition is managed properly, there is no reason why you cannot engage in sporting activity at any time of the year. You just have to be a lot more careful than someone without asthma.

Preventing exercise-induced asthma

It might seem that the simplest way to prevent exercise-induced asthma is to be a lazy slob and to do no exercise at all. But that would merely make stress-related attacks more probable, as well as significantly raising your chances of having heart disease, obesity-linked diabetes and arthritis! There are better ways of preventing exercise-induced asthma than putting the rest of your health at risk.

The first step is to make quite sure that your treatment is right. Daily Peak Expiratory Flow (PEF) readings will help you to see when your asthma is worsening. Also, make sure you use your inhalers properly; if you have any doubts at all, ask to see your practice nurse for advice. Take steps to reduce stress, have a nutritious diet and follow any other courses you think you need to keep your asthma under control.

People with well controlled asthma only very rarely suffer exercise-induced attacks. Almost all exercise-induced asthma appears in people whose condition is not being properly controlled. And all the evidence so far points to the fact that people with poorly controlled asthma are not doing what the doctor ordered. They are "forgetting" some treatments, or not using the inhaler properly, or simply ignoring what the doctor says. Exercise-induced attacks can be avoided by most sufferers if they take their treatments properly.

Planning for exercise

Almost everyone with asthma can take part in exercise, providing they plan their activity and prepare themselves properly.

If your condition is already well-controlled by medication, you should first consider what kind of exercise to take. Cross country running in the middle of winter is not always a good idea – for the cold air can trigger an attack even in people who are pretty good at controlling their disease. However, with care, it can be done. You just need to think about how much you want to go cross country running in winter and the risks of having an attack. A discussion with your doctor about your own individual circumstances is a good idea before you take up any sport.

Once you have settled on the form of sport or exercise that most appeals to you, get some training. Don't just launch into cross country running, or downhill skiing without some preparation. Not only will you be more likely to suffer an injury, but you will also exert more effort than necessary and put extra strain on your lungs.

Use your inhaler immediately before the exercise. This will have the effect of opening up your airways and making any problems induced by cold air less troublesome.

Some athletes find that they can bring on exercise-induced wheezing during their warm up, only to find that they do not suffer any chest trouble at all, half an hour later in actual competition. If this happens to you, your exercise regime may need to include a warm up period that induces chest wheeziness as a way of avoiding more serious discomfort later.

Studies have shown that a series of brief sprints, lasting for about 30 seconds each over a five minute period, can be very effective in preventing exercise-induced attacks.

Which exercise?

There are few exercises that people with asthma cannot do. No matter what the sport may be, almost anyone with asthma can do it.

However, some forms of exercise do bring on more attacks than others. Running, for some unknown reason, appears high on the list of those that trigger attacks of asthma. Curiously, cycling is much less of a problem.

Exercise-induced asthma is extremely variable. You may discover that you can take part in basketball with no problem, but find cricket difficult. Only by trial and error are you likely to find a form of exercise you enjoy that does not trigger attacks of asthma.

Try wearing a scarf over your mouth and nose if you must exercise in cold air. It will warm the air slightly as you breathe in and make an attack of asthma less likely.

Swimming

Swimming is the best exercise for people with asthma. Indeed, there are special swimming clubs all over the country for asthma sufferers.

It seems that the warm, moist air does the reverse of cold dry air. Instead of irritating the linings of the airways, it soothes them. This should come as no surprise as a steam inhalation is one of the mainstays of treating a bad cold. The warm moist air relieves the blocked-up nasal passages by soothing them.

In addition to helping your lungs, swimming is a good all-round exercise that uses virtually every muscle in your body. So it helps with your general health and fitness.

Exercise-induced attacks

Some people only get asthma attacks after exercise. At other times, they breathe normally and have no signs or symptoms of the disease. This can be worrying for them as they often first suspect that the exercise has brought on a heart attack or some very serious problem. However, they usually recover within a few minutes – demonstrating the power of cold air to irritate the lining of the airways.

If you have exercise-induced asthma, your doctor is likely to want to test your breathing to find out what is going on and how bad the problem is in your case. This means you may well need to perform some breathing tests in a hospital laboratory. Then you will be asked to exercise, usually on a treadmill machine, before further breathing tests. The tests will probably be repeated again after treatment. This kind of testing helps to establish the right level of treatment for you to prevent such attacks.

Even so, exercise-induced asthma does vary. The exercise you perform one day might not lead to symptoms. But on another day, less severe exercise might bring on an attack.

Attacks are also influenced by the length of time you exercise. Research has shown that you need to exercise for about eight minutes or more to bring on more than generalised wheezing. But exercising for longer than eight minutes does not increase the severity of an attack.

Most exercise-induced attacks occur within fifteen minutes of exercising. But some individuals can get a second attack between four and ten hours after stopping exercise. Quite why this occurs is as yet unexplained; but it does happen to about one in every three people who suffer from exercise-induced asthma.

Exercise and hay fever

The biggest problem for hay fever sufferers who like exercise is that playing in the big outdoors is likely to bring them into contact with pollens. This is particularly true since most people take part in sporting activity during the spring and summer months. It seems that only the truly dedicated play sports in winter.

If you suffer from hay fever and want to enjoy the benefits of exercise, you clearly have a problem if you want to go walking in the country or hiking or even playing football on a newly-mown pitch. To avoid problems, you should try to find out which pollen is the cause of your symptoms.

Your doctor can test for the particular allergen by using a special skin test. If this test discovers that a grass pollen is to blame for your symptoms, you need to consider an outdoor activity that keeps you away from grass. That's difficult; but an all-weather athletics tracks might be possible – or you could play tennis, using a hard court.

If your hay fever is due to a particular tree pollen, you can avoid any sport that takes you close to such trees. Or you can avoid playing outdoor games at particular times of the year.

Tree pollens occur at specific times of the year – though there may be some variation from year to year because of weather and climatic changes. April and May are the worst months, since this is when most trees pollinate.

So, exercising indoors in the spring may be better for people who have hay fever associated with tree pollen. For this reason tennis is a good idea. You can play on indoor courts in the winter and spring, only venturing outside in the summer after most trees have pollinated.

If your hay fever is due to grass pollens, playing outdoors in the summer is not a good idea as the air is full of grass pollen from May to September. You might consider swimming, as this will give you good all-round exercise and the warm moist air of an indoor pool will help soothe your nose and throat.

Exercise programmes

It is a good idea to have an exercise programme, whether you suffer from asthma or hay fever. You will not derive the full benefit from exercise if you only do it occasionally.

Exercise will keep you fit. It will improve your general health and boost your immune system if you suffer from allergies. All this means that regular, well planned exercise is an essential part of keeping your condition in check.

Ideally, you should have three main periods of exercise each week. These need only last 20 minutes each; but if you don't plan for them, they won't happen! Studies have shown that you get more benefit from three 20 minute periods of exercise than from a single hour.

If possible, try to exercise on weekdays when most people go to work, come home and then sit in front of the TV all evening! People tend to be more active at weekends with shopping, gardening and the like.

Try to keep as active as possible in addition to your three periods of regular exercise. This means walking to the local shop rather than taking the car for the one mile trip. Use the stairs, rather than lifts or escalators. Get off the bus a stop early and walk the rest of the way. Do anything that makes you more active physically. All such activity is beneficial. Combined with the three periods of more structured exercise each week, it will make you feel healthier and enable you to handle your symptoms more easily.

Chapter 12
Some Special Problems

Holidays

Everyone likes holidays – well almost everyone. People with asthma and hay fever often find them somewhat problematic.

Holidays can be ruined for someone with asthma or hay fever. Without knowing it, you can find yourself holidaying in a region where the allergen that triggers your condition is in plentiful supply. You will then spend your entire holiday in misery, suffering from symptoms most of the time.

You can still have problems on holiday even if your condition is not caused by an allergy. Asthma triggered by cold air can be a problem for those who holiday on the coast in countries with a cold climate. Cool breezes might feel refreshing; but breathing in these conditions may lead to asthma symptoms.

Choosing a holiday destination

Choose somewhere that doesn't have the allergen that triggers your symptoms. If you are allergic to pine trees, for instance, don't plan a holiday in the spring in Florida where these species are prevalent. You can find out which trees are common in particular areas by asking travel agents and local tourist boards.

For people with asthma, a coastal holiday is often ideal since the air is humid and soothes irritable lungs. Good destinations for people with asthma are areas where the humidity is relatively high, though not oppressive, and where the weather is warm. The Mediterranean coastline is a good place to consider.

Pollen counts are lowest around coastlines, thanks to conditions that cause the air to be blown inland. No pollen come from the sea and so the air that pushes inwards is pollen free. Hence hay fever also is much less likely at seaside resorts.

Deciding when to go

The time of year chosen for a holiday is much more important to people with hay fever and asthma than for people who do not have these conditions. If you have hay fever caused by a particular pollen, you do not want to go away and spend a great deal of time outdoors when this pollen is in full flight. If grass pollen is your problem, July and August are not a good time to go away.

People with asthma also find that their condition worsens in the winter months when the cold dry air irritates the lining of their airways. Hence a winter sunshine holiday can be ideal. Going to a coastal resort in the Canaries or the Mediterranean may be just the tonic needed by someone with asthma during a cold British winter.

What kind of holiday?

Almost any kind of holiday will do, providing it is at a suitable time of the year and well away from allergens.

Why not consider a cruise if you can afford it. At sea, you will be well away from the vast majority of allergens that trigger asthma and hay fever. Indeed, there are no pollens to get up your nose out at sea.

Try to avoid certain types of holidays, such as camping, which bring you into close contact with pollens and dusts that can lead to symptoms. Also, people with asthma may find that skiing holidays are not much fun as the cold air can trigger attacks.

Flying

One of the biggest worries for people with asthma is flying to foreign destinations. There are two principal concerns. One is the fear that if they have an attack six miles above the surface of the earth, medical help is a long way away; this causes tremendous anxiety and fear in some sufferers. The other concern is that the pressurisation of the cabin can trigger attacks.

An aircraft cabin is pressurised to the same atmospheric pressure as that at an altitude of about six thousand feet. This is the happy medium that prevents the aircraft's structure from breaking apart. This is not a major problem for people with asthma. If you do have an attack – often brought on by being stressed – you will find that the cabin crew is well trained to cope. Not only do its members have high levels of medical skills, but every aircraft carries oxygen cylinders for use in emergencies. Also, cabin crew rarely have to ask if there is a doctor on board – they know from the passenger list.

So flying is not a problem for people with asthma. Only if you have very severe, chronic asthma should you seek advice from your doctor before flying and let the airline know so that any necessary special arrangements can be made.

House dust mites

You can take every precaution at home to rid yourself of house dust mites, but you can be sure that they will be in your hotel room or apartment when you arrive in your holiday destination. Clearly, your asthma could come on quickly if you have spent much of your time in a well-cleaned, dust mite free environment at home.

It is not practical to take special vacuum cleaners and humidifiers away with you on holiday. However, you can pack your mattress covers (if you use them). Then you will at least limit your contact with the dust mites.

You might also consider anti-dust mite sprays for holidays. You can get these sprays from your local pharmacy. They work by attacking the droppings of the house dust mite and rendering them harmless. You can treat your hotel room with spray and thus avoid contact with the allergen – helping you to enjoy your holiday. Some people use these sprays at home; but if you take good effective action against the dust mites, you probably don't need the sprays as well.

Planning for a holiday

You need to consider holidays more carefully when you have asthma or hay fever; and you obviously must plan effectively. But planning requires more than just decision-making about where and when to go.

You need to be sure that you have enough medication with you to last throughout the time you are away from home. Be sure to visit your GP in plenty of time to get the relevant prescriptions. Drugs are different in each country; and getting precisely what you need for your asthma or hay fever may not be possible where you are staying. So, stock up in advance.

Also, make quite sure that your holiday insurance has proper cover.

Many holiday insurance policies will not cover you for "pre-existing" conditions. Also some policies specifically exclude cover for expenses incurred as a result of asthma attacks. Read the small print of your holiday insurance policy and if necessary seek the advice of an independent insurance broker. The last thing you would want after a holiday ruined by a severe asthma attack is a huge bill for the medical care.

Be sure to complete the form E111 if you are going to a country within the European Union. This form allows you to get free healthcare treatment on holiday. Forms can be obtained from your travel agent.

On holiday

When you arrive at your destination make sure you know where to get medical help should you need it. This should be one of the first things you do after arrival. You probably will not need help; but it's better to know, just in case.

Have a look round to check whether there are any potential allergens. For example, ask to have your room changed if you find a tree growing outside your bedroom window. This is made easier by many holiday companies if you have specifically mentioned your health problem on the booking form.

Once in your room, spray the bed and the furnishings with anti-dust mite spray before putting on your anti-allergy bed covers. Then relax and enjoy your holiday – you don't want to have stress-induced attacks of symptoms.

Work

Going to work can be a real problem for people with hay fever or asthma. Imagine having to travel into work on a hot summer's day when the air is full of pollen. By the time you get to the office, your eyes are streaming, your nose is running and your throat feels dry and sore. Working under those conditions can be very difficult.

Similarly, what if it's a clear, cold morning in winter. A stiff wind could bring on wheezing for people with asthma. They then have to face a day at the workbench, wheezing, inhaling and hoping to avoid an attack.

Neither scenario is likely to make working an enjoyable experience.

Avoiding trouble at work

The best policy is honesty. Let your boss know that you have asthma or hay fever and that certain weather conditions may mean that it is best for you to stay at home.

Explain that you will be well – providing you stay at home; but that you may fall ill if you venture out. An understanding boss will realise the benefit of keeping indoors under particular conditions. If you go in to work you will be less than fully productive for a number of days – rather than just for the single day you have off.

But your chances of taking time off will be much reduced if you do not explain the problem in advance.

Choosing the right job

If possible, choose a job in the right location, away from things that cause your symptoms.

That's not always easy, particularly if you have only just developed symptoms and you have been with the company for a number of years. However, you may be able to transfer to another part of the firm to avoid symptoms and be more efficient.

When applying for new jobs, take a good look at the surroundings. Are the offices surrounded by grass that could be a problem in the summer if you have hay fever? Are there plants in the offices that might produce a pollen which affects you? Are there heavy plush carpets that will be a breeding ground for dust mites? Consider all this kind of thing before accepting a new job.

If you really want the job and anything like this troubles you, discuss it with your potential employer. Something can usually be worked out to minimise your symptoms.

Occupational asthma

Some people develop asthma for the first time when they start a new job – even though the symptoms might take many months to develop. Others who have mild asthma find that their condition is worsened considerably by their occupation. You can tell if this is the case if your symptoms are bad during the week but are mild or non-existent at weekends.

Asthma linked to a job – occupational asthma – is relatively common.

Many people find that they become wheezy at work; and there are certain industries which are renowned for causing chest complaints. Often these involve processes which use chemicals or produce large clouds of dust.

Manufacturing companies that make foam or detergents can have employees who develop asthma as a direct result of the chemicals used. Those who work in bakeries or mills are also more prone to asthma because of the clouds of dust involved. Pharmaceutical manufacturing can also be linked to asthma as can laboratory work.

The UK Government has now accepted that occupational asthma is a real problem. Consequently, there is a compensation scheme for people who develop occupational asthma. To gain compensation, you need to be able to show that a particular allergen has caused your symptoms and that this allergen is used in your place of work. It's not as complicated as it sounds. Your GP and your local office of the Department of Social Security can help you make your case.

Once you have applied for compensation, you will need to attend a special hearing and be examined by two doctors who do not know you. Your own doctor will also be required to provide evidence.

The compensation you receive is not fixed and depends upon a number of different factors. You can apply for an increase if you believe your asthma has worsened.

Pregnancy

Women with asthma often worry that their asthma will worsen when they become pregnant – or that it will endanger the baby.

They also worry that the drugs used can harm the growing baby. Then there are further worries that a difficult labour could induce an asthma attack – just at the wrong moment.

Fortunately, all those concerns are easily dismissed. Hardly any women have trouble with pregnancy or childbirth as a direct result of asthma. Also, the vast majority of the drugs used in asthma are safe and highly unlikely to harm the growing baby. Most of the drugs are inhaled anyway. They work only in the lungs and never reach the baby. Even if a woman is taking steroid tablets, there is little risk to the baby from the low doses most doctors prescribe.

Occasionally, pregnant women find that the baby needs more oxygen in the later stages of pregnancy – which forces the mother to breathe more to meet the demand. This can be a problem with very severe asthma and may make the mother's symptoms worse. Fortunately, such cases are very rare indeed.

Labour itself is never a problem. The hormones released in labour help to dampen down the asthma, so the chances of an attack are naturally much lessened.

Nocturnal asthma

One particularly troublesome fact about asthma is its tendency to produce symptoms in the middle of the night. Three out of every four people with asthma are awakened every now and then by symptoms during the night. The most common time is 4 am.

The reasons for this nocturnal asthma are not completely understood. Part of the problem appears to be a natural variation in the size of our airways at night. During the night everyone's airways narrow down a little; but if you have asthma, this natural occurrence can cause real difficulties.

The trouble is that most people with asthma accept as normal their waking in the night with breathing problems. It isn't normal. Waking at night as a result of asthma shows that the condition is not under complete control. "Normal" people never wake up wheezing in the early hours of the morning.

Even those who have good daytime control of their asthma can wake up at night because of symptoms. This means they may need additional drugs specifically to control the night-time symptoms. Or they may need their daytime dosage to be altered to provide extra protection throughout the night.

So, if you have asthma and you wake during the night, don't accept that as normal. See your GP and you will probably be given treatment to help your airways to open and to prevent wheezing. That way you will get a good night's rest.

Chapter 13
A Complete Plan for
Dealing with Asthma and Hay Fever

Both asthma and hay fever can be improved by following a few common steps. These will achieve a reduction in symptoms and less severe attacks if they do arise.

Step 1

The first thing to do is get medical advice if you have any trouble at all with breathing or any kind of irritation to your lungs, throat, nose or eyes.

It's no good thinking the problem is minor. It probably won't go away and you could be increasing the chances of danger in the future.

Step 2

Follow the doctor's advice. Learn how to take the treatment properly.

If you have an asthma inhaler, get proper advice from your practice nurse. If you have nose drops for hay fever, take them properly so the drugs get to where they are needed. You will only get full benefit from medicines if you take them as they are supposed to be taken.

If you have asthma, make a visit to an asthma clinic a regular part of your care. Also be sure to follow the clinic's instructions and use a Peak Flow Meter to monitor your condition.

Step 3

Try to find out what triggers the symptoms. The chances are it is the droppings of house dust mites, grass pollen or particular foods.

Keep a diary of your symptoms, your activities and your food intake. Try to match episodes of symptoms with the activities you undertook and the food you ate. This will give a big clue to the cause of your symptoms.

You should ask your doctor about allergy tests; in some cases they are helpful in pinpointing the cause.

Step 4

Once you have found out what triggers your symptoms, avoid those activities or foods if possible.

This may mean changing your diet or altering your lifestyle. It may involve taking action to remove dust mites from your house, or certain plants and grasses from your garden. It may even mean moving house. The aim is to avoid contact with the particular factor that causes your symptoms.

Step 5

Reduce stress in your life. Learn to manage your time effectively. Learn relaxation and breathing techniques to help calm your nerves. Take up a creative hobby. In fact do anything that takes your mind off your condition and makes you feel better in yourself.

Step 6

Get regular exercise. Preferably go swimming three times a week for 20 minutes at a time. Or take three brisk walks each week. Become more active. Use stairs instead of lifts.

If your symptoms are brought on by exercise, take your medication in advance. If exercising brings you into contact with the things that cause your symptoms, choose another kind of exercise.

Step 7

Change your diet. Consider a diet that is rich in fibre and has plenty of vitamins and minerals in it – particularly Vitamin B12. Also avoid foods that contain the E numbers E220 to E227.

You may need to take vitamin and mineral supplements if you have a busy life and do not eat regular meals with plenty of fresh fruit and vegetables.

Step 8

Don't keep your condition a secret. Tell people who need to know, such as employers, teachers, relatives and so on. Any one of them may need to act if you have a severe attack of symptoms.

They can also be of help if symptoms develop and there is something practical they can do to make your work or education more comfortable.

Step 9

Keep an eye on the weather. Watch the TV weather bulletins, or catch up on them on the radio or in the newspapers. This will help you find out if each day is going to produce the conditions that will lead to symptoms.

Listen especially for the air quality figures – the pollen count and the wind chill factor. Either of these can trigger symptoms. By listening to the weather you may be able to re-plan your day so as to avoid coming into contact with things that cause trouble.

Step 10

Consider alternative medicine. Many of the herbal and homeopathic remedies can help.

Tell your doctor that you are considering supplementing the orthodox treatment with extra assistance from alternative therapies. Many people with asthma and hay fever find that these non-traditional sources of medical and health advice are a real boon.

However, never interrupt or cease orthodox medical treatment in favour of alternative remedies unless your doctor tells you that it is safe to do so. Otherwise you could be putting yourself at extreme risk.

Summary

Following these steps can help you to keep your asthma or hayfever under control and allow you to lead a normal life without being too encumbered by your condition.

However, everyone is different. The only person who can really advise you is the person who knows most about your medical history and your specific circumstances – your GP. Your own doctor is central to your care. Consequently the above advice, and indeed the whole contents of this book, should be considered as supplementary to what your doctor might say.

Chapter 14
The National Asthma Campaign

The National Asthma Campaign (NAC) is Britain's leading charity dedicated to help every aspect of asthma. It also helps in the field of hay fever. The NAC was formed by the merger of the Asthma Research Council, the Friends of the Asthma Research Council, and the Asthma Society, separate organisations which joined together in 1990 to form a single body.

The NAC works in three principal areas. It funds research into asthma and allergy. It provides benefits and services for people with asthma. And it has an educational role, spreading knowledge about asthma and its treatment.

Research

The research funded by the NAC is performed at a number of different hospitals and universities in the UK. Researchers have to submit their plans to the NAC which then decides whether funding should be provided. In 1993 the charity spent £1.9m on research – more than any other non-commercial organisation, including the government.

Help and mutual support

The NAC has a range of newspapers, leaflets and books to help people with asthma. It also holds local branch meetings where people with asthma, or their parents, can get together. These offer mutual support and also allow you to learn more about the condition. There are 180 branches in the UK and meetings are usually attended by a doctor who can explain medical matters if necessary.

The NAC also provides a nationwide information line. The Asthma Helpline is run from 1pm to 9pm each weekday. The telephone calls are charged at local rates, no matter where you dial from. The number is 0345 010203.

There is a Junior Asthma Club, for children aged between seven and twelve, which has its own newsletter with information especially designed for youngsters.

Education

The NAC also campaigns on issues and helps improve services for people with asthma. One of its specific projects has been to improve the understanding of teachers. The NAC has produced a special Schools Pack which provides posters and a step by step guide explaining what teachers should do if one of their pupils has an attack.

To find out more about the National Asthma Campaign write to or telephone the organisation:

National Asthma Campaign,
Providence House, Providence Place, London N1 0NT.
Telephone 071-226 2260. Fax 071-704 0740.

You could also try contacting your local branch. Your GP or your local public library will have the telephone number.

A selection of other titles from Imperia Books

You Can Beat Arthritis

"This is an excellent book – and much overdue. It should have a place on the bookshelf in every home." *Dr Ann Robinson*

Too many people put up with the pain of arthritis unaware of the options now available to them. This book explains all the medical and alternative remedies successful in treating arthritis, rheumatism and related back pain.

The book provides fresh insight into the conditions which aggravate arthritis, explains how these can be remedied and reveals the key to a greatly improved quality of life. The message throughout the book is one of hope.

Price £11.95 inclusive of postage and handling

£500 A Week From Car Boot Sales

This insider's guide tells all there is to know about successful car booting. It lifts the lid off the booting phenomenon and exposes the massive profits being made weekly in the big money spinner of the 1990s.

The book reveals how to obtain stock for next to nothing, how to find the best pitches and sell at 1000% profit. It also shows how to turn browsers into buyers and discloses ways of telling real antiques from junk.

Buyers, novice booters and even experienced sellers will be amazed by Roger Morgan's account of all the tricks of the trade – the cons, the frauds, the fakes and the selling and buying ploys one would never even dream of.

Price £9.95 inclusive of postage and handling

1,717 Natural Healing Remedies (Kulopathy)

This book reveals many vital remedies based on natural and alternative medicines. It also tells how to detect and overcome the nutritional deficiencies which cause bad health.

Here is just a small selection of the many remedies contained in the book:

8 ways to combat arthritis • 6 remedies for incontinence and other bladder problems • 4 treatments for prostate disorders • 3 ways to reduce breathlessness • 4 ways of overcoming impotence • 3 suggestions to lower blood pressure • A simple treatment to relieve piles • 4 remedies for bad indigestion • 7 suggestions for poor sleepers

Price £9.95 inclusive of postage and handling

How To Find Your Ideal Partner

This book is for the millions of unattached people, whether single, divorced or widowed, who hope one day to form a close loving relationship with an ideal partner.

Readers are shown how to develop a greater understanding of themselves and the type of partner they are seeking. Many different methods of meeting a potential partner are explored – from leisure activities to introduction agencies, from singles clubs to personal ads.

The author also gives helpful, practical advice on how to create the right impression and build a relationship from the first date to a long term commitment.

Price £9.95 inclusive of postage and handling

Quest For The Messiah

This book tells the fascinating story of Man's constant struggle to create a paradise on earth.

Throughout history, self-professed messiahs arose again and again in response to biblical prophesies whenever human suffering reached a new peak. These ranged from saints and pious simpletons to megalomaniac tricksters. The terrible struggles of their followers from the time of Jesus to the present day makes fascinating reading.

Scrupulously researched, Quest for the Messiah is the story of the highest human aspirations and the curious mixture of genuine piety, sex, violence and sheer evil that so often resulted. It is an enthralling story – and a true one!

Price £9.95 inclusive of postage and handling

The Hard of Hearing Handbook

"This is an excellent book – and much overdue. It is essential reading for everyone with a deaf friend, acquaintance, colleague or member of the family." *The Rt. Hon. Alfred Morris MP, formerly Minister for the Disabled*

The world of those who cannot hear well can easily become isolated and bleak; but this book shows that it need not be so. The book highlights the dozens of ways in which practical help can be made available and reveals how to cope with the emotional and everyday problems of hearing disability.

For well-meaning people, who often find themselves at a loss when attempting to talk to those who do not hear well, this book has an important role. It explains how to make small adjustments which can make a huge difference to the hard of hearing and enable them to remain fully in touch with the world around them.

Price £11.95 inclusive of postage and handling

Ordering

To order any of the above books, please send your name, address, book titles required and payment (cheque/P.O. or Visa/Access number and expiry date) to Imperia Books Limited, P O Box 191, Edgware, Middlesex HA8 7NY.

Please allow 7 to 21 days for delivery. A full refund will be given for books returned within 28 days.